Food, Herbs, Health, & Healing

John E. Smith
B.A.(Hons.) M:URHP Dip.C.H.

Strategic Book Publishing
New York, New York

Strategic Book Publishing
An imprint of Writers Literary & Publishing Services, Inc.
845 Third Avenue, 6th Floor – 6016
New York, NY 10022
http://www.strategicbookpublishing.com

ISBN: 978-1-60860-653-5

Printed in the United States of America

Book Design: Suzanne Kelly

To all the great proponents of every healing tradition and to my teachers, past, present, and future.

Acknowledgments

MY THANKS GO TO my teachers:
Michael Tierra L.Ac., O.M.D.
Dr. David Frawley,
Hakeem G.M. Chishti,
Maharishi Mahesh Yogi,
Dr. J. Naidu.

For patience and willingness to read through the first draft, my wife, Jenny.

For efficiency, patience, and technical advice, my thanks to the staff of Strategic Books.

Disclaimer

ANY HEALTH BENEFITS CITED IN this text are based on centuries of traditional herbal use and not, unless specified, on modern scientific findings.

The information contained in this book is for educational purposes and is not intended as an alternative to the advice of a qualified health practitioner.

Table of Contents

John E. Smith

Preface

So where do I start?

Do I start from the seed? —No I came much earlier.

Do I start from the root (radix—the beginning)?

No! —I was once a rootless vagrant, floating in seas of primordial soup.

An alga, a one celled nutrient.

It was many millennia before I attached myself to rock, created earth, and grew to inhabit, and become, the swamps, the forests, and the mountain.

I remember well the coming of Behemoth, the giant reptiles, the woolly mammoth,

The hairy men learning to stand erect, to burn me on their fires,

And drink me, to drive away parasites.

Who am I?

I am the power of healing

I am the Earth maker, the ground shaker

I am Ambrotus, Soma, Isis, Gaia

I am Chiron, Aesclupius, Gabriel

I am essence, spirit, Ruh, Shen—the messengers of heaven

I have been with you from the dawn of your day,

And when you are poisoned by your own stupidity,

I will be there to pass on the keys to the next tenants.

Introduction

IN MY EARLIER BOOK, *100 Herbs of Power* (Strategic Book Publishing, New York 2008), I covered fifty to sixty herbs in reasonable depth and introduced another fifty or so. These are all key herbs, used in natural medicine by various traditions. It is not my intention to cover these herbs again in this text; although many of them will be referred to in passing.

There are literally millions of plants used, as either foods or medicines, and many of these will be featured in this book, together with some traditional formulations, combinations, simple recipes, and healing strategies.

The aim of holistic medicine is to support the harmonious functioning of mind, body, and spirit, to create or maintain a state of homeostasis, whereas allopathic medicine aims to change the problematic expression of a particular function. In allopathic medicine the prefix "anti" occurs often, and if you think about it, some of the "anti" words actually infer a serious negative, e.g., "antibiotic" translates as "against life."

Technically speaking, herbalists and practitioners of natural medicine are not allowed by law to make claims regarding a particular herb or medicine; the best we can do is use phrases such as "will support a healthy immune system." I have, however, used terms such as antibiotic, anti-inflammatory, etc., with regard to many herbs as these are correct terms and easy to relate to by the modern western reader. The Chinese may use terms such as "combat external evils" or "drain fire," and in Ayurveda, terms such as "reduce ama" (stagnation) or "calm pitta" (fire) may abound, and I have used these terms where appropriate.

Another difference with the recording of allopathic and natural medicines is that chemical drugs will usually fall into

1

particular categories, whereas herbs often have many different functions; e.g., hawthorn, generally known as a heart tonic, will also relieve indigestion caused by food stagnation. Again, for simplicity I have listed many herbs under their most relevant organ system.

In traditional Chinese Medicine, listings would include such headings as "herbs to tonify qi" or "herbs to reduce damp," but the same problem may arise in that a herb such as Atractylodes will perform both of these functions; so even these headings become restricting.

Western allopathic medicine bases all of its findings on scientific research, which unfortunately is far from conclusive. We have seen how "well researched" and licensed medicines have created major health problems, and it has been cited many times how research laboratories are largely funded by pharmaceutical concerns, so research projects, rather like statistics, can show what we want them to show depending on our particular bias. Research has been carried out regarding many herbs, giving all manner of different results. Homeopathy has been "proven" to be ineffective regardless of the millions who benefit from its use, and herbal medicine is generally considered by the establishment to be potentially dangerous, regardless of the fact that there are fewer deaths from medicinal herbs than there are from the humble potato, and prescribed, licensed medicines kill ten times the number of people killed by knives and firearms combined. So, my apologies for not citing too many research references; they do exist, but to be honest I don't find them very relevant. I prefer to trust in traditional usage and feel that if a plant has been used successfully for a few hundred, (or in some cases a few thousand) years that makes it safer than something that has just been created by a powerful pharmaceutical giant. But that is my personal bias.

In my earlier book, my chapter headings related to different health systems, e.g., Chinese Medicine, Ayurveda, and Western Herbalism, etc. I have used a similar approach in this volume, but the herbs listed under the section relating to the Chinese Five Element organ systems will often contains herbs from

India, Europe, and other cultures. Again specific listings can be problematic, e.g., to list ginger under Ayurvedic rather than Chinese or even Western herbalism could be considered incorrect. Many herbs considered as Western may be used or grown in the East and vice-versa. Dandelion is commonly used in China, as is American Ginseng. In my practice I will generally combine herbs from several traditions in one formula. It is my hope that readers of this book will gain some benefits from its pages.

CHAPTER ONE

The Folklore and History of Natural Medicine

AESCLEPIUS, THE GREEK GOD OF healing was supposedly born of a union between a woman and a god; he was killed and became divine. The tradition of Aesclepius started around 2000 B.C.

The Greek tradition of Medicine was championed by Hippocrates "The Father of Medicine" (460–373 B.C.) and his later followers, Theophrastus (371–287 B.C.) who wrote *Enquiry into Plants and the Causes of Plants*, Dioscorides (50–70 A.D.) who wrote the first Western Materia Medica, and Galen (131–201 A.D.) who became the personal physician of the Emperor Marcus Aurelius.

The legends of natural healing in ancient India go back to "The Golden Age of India" to the time of the Indus Valley civilization (approx 2,600 B.C.) and beyond to the great epic legends of the Vedas (see the chapter on Ayurveda).

Chinese legends take us back to the great legendary Emperors Shen Nong and Huang Di who lived between 5000 and 2000 B.C. Shen Nong (the Agricultural Emperor) was thought to have had a transparent body through which he could view the actions of the herbs he imbibed. Huang Di (The Yellow Emperor) is generally considered to be responsible for the great systems of Chinese Medicine (including acupuncture). The two great texts of Chinese medicine *Shen Nong Ben Cao Jing* (The Divine Farmer's Herb Root Classic) and *Huangdi Neijing* (The Yellow Emperor's Classic of Internal Medicine) were compiled much later, sometime in the Han Dynasty (202 B.C.–220 A.D.)

In the ninth century A.D. The Kurdish Botanist Al Dinawari (826–896 A.D.) published his *Book of Plants (Kitab al Nabat)*. One century later Avicenna (Ibn Sina) produced his great *Canon of Medicine* and *Book of Healing (Kitab al Shifa)*.

Physicians such as Culpepper and Gerard have continued these traditions of plant-based medicine to the modern day.

Homeostatsis

"The constancy of the internal environment is the condition for a free and independent life"
—Claude Bernard (1813–1878)

In all traditions Mother Nature is seen as a healing goddess (Bhumi Devi in India, Gaia and Hygea in Ancient Greece, etc.) and the function of nature is to achieve and maintain a state of balance, equilibrium, and homeostasis. Early physicians such as Hippocrates saw the role of the "healer" as being the servant or facilitator of nature in maintaining this state of homeostasis. This underlying principle is inherent in the teachings of Aristotle (384–322 B.C.), Epicurius (341–270 B.C.), Caraka (First century A.D.), and Avicenna (Tenth century A.D.).

Iraq was a pivotal point in bringing ancient wisdom to the modern world. A ninth century Caliph of Baghdad once dreamed of being visited by the ancient Greek scholar Aristotle and as a result encouraged the translation of the works of the earliest Greek philosophers into Arabic. Many of his contemporaries, including Avicenna, encouraged the revival of ancient Greek wisdom, which spread throughout Arabic culture. Avicenna took this further and included not only the teachings of Hippocrates but also those of Eastern physicians including Charak and Susrut, together with the medical teachings of ancient Persia in his *Canon of Medicine* and *The Book of Healing. The Canon of Medicine* was translated into Mandarin in 1659 under the heading *Prescriptions of the Hui Nationality.* The texts of Ibn Sina (Avicenna) are still taught in UCLA and Yale University, and they are of primary importance in Unani Tibb medicine, a principle healing philosophy throughout the middle and Far East.

In the nineteenth century physicians such as Pasteur, Fleming, Jenner, etc., became fixated with the concept of bacteria and viruses, a concept that dominates modern medicine with its preoccupation with antibiotics, antivirals, and suppressant drugs.

Claude Bernard (1813–1878) disagreed strongly with Pasteur, who laid the blame for sickness on bacteria, stating that:

"The microbe is nothing, the terrain is everything."

Thereby reiterating the importance of the concept of homeostasis, or maintaining balance within and without the individual.

According to certain sources[1] Louis Pasteur on his deathbed conceded that Claude Bernard was right.

Wholeness

Health is not just an absence of disease but a state of wholeness. The word "health" comes from the old English word "haelth" meaning "whole." Haelth in turn comes from the German root "hal" meaning health, happiness, and wholeness; the word "holiness" comes from the same root, as of course does the word "holistic."

The body is not just a collection of organs working independently, but a synergy of differing connected energies, which create wholeness. Holistic medicine treats the person from this premise. Perfect health is a state of perfect balance between body, mind, emotions, spirit, and environment. Although we are all individual, we are all made up of the same elements and energies; these may be in different proportions according to our constitution or body type, and therefore we may need different considerations. As Hippocrates the father of Western medicine said:

"It is more important to know what kind of person has the disease than what kind of disease a person has."

For it is only then that we can attempt to create or maintain balance.

"Every individual organism that has a distinctive genetic background has distinctive nutritional needs, which must be met for optimal well-being."
—Roger Williams

All traditional systems of medicine agree on these concepts even if philosophies differ, parallels can generally be made, and balance is always the aim of holistic medicine.

A strong thread of this concept of health as wholeness exists right up until the more dualistic teachings of western philosophers, such as Descartes and the later medical specialists who wished to divide the body up (often literally) into various parts, which are often considered in isolation, rather than as part of a whole.

CHAPTER TWO

External Considerations

"The sibyl of Cumae was granted long life by the God Apollo. She was allowed as many years as the grains that she was able to hold in one hand. Carelessly the sibyl forgot to ask for eternal youth. She became ugly with age and her prophetic powers declined. In later life, when asked what she wanted most, she replied, 'I want to die.'"

Taken from *The Satyricon*—
Petronius, first century A.D.

General Bodycare

CARE OF THE TEETH: Clean with fingers using herbal powders mixed with sesame oil and salt.

Suggested Formula: catechu, rock salt, black pepper, turmeric, neem (equal parts) with a drop of myrrh tincture, a few drops of honey, and sufficient sesame oil to form a paste.

CARE OF MOUTH: Gargle with one tablespoon of warm sesame oil, with the addition of one or two drops of myrrh tincture.

CARE OF TONGUE: Scraping with stainless steel, silver, or bamboo tongue scraper.

CARE OF NASAL PASSAGES: (Nasya) A few drops of Brahmi oil or Brahmi ghee into each nostril at night. Vinegar with rose water is a good alternative.

CARE OF THE THROAT: Gargle with decoction of sumac and red clover or Usnea and goldenseal. Sea salt makes a simple basis for a soothing gargle, as does colloidal silver.

CARE OF THE EYES: Exercising the eyes is very important in improving vision. Moving the pupils up and down, from left to right, from a focus on a distant horizon to an observation of a nearby object, and viewing different colours in the environment, will all help to expand and contract the pupils, giving them a visual "work out." Light massage over the eyelids, with the fingertips will also be useful.

There are certain herbs taken internally that are known to improve vision; they include: Shatavari (Indian Asparagus Root), Schizandra fruit, Eyebright herb, Lycium (Goji berries), and Solomon's seal root. Eyebright can be used as a weak tea in eyebaths.

A highly recommended Chinese Tea Formula for the eyes is made up from equal parts of Lycii berries (Goji), He Shou Wu (P.multiflorum), Red Jujube dates, and Chrysanthemum flowers (C.morifolium). Fifty grams of this mixture is simmered in a litre of water in a covered pot for 20–30 minutes, strained, and drunk over two days. This should be repeated frequently. These ingredients are included in the formula "Bright Eye Shining Pill."[2]

HEALING BATHS: Echinacea leaves, Marigold petals, Rose Petals, and Elderflowers (a tablespoon of each) together with one tablespoon of Infused Calendula Oil (not essential oil, which would be too strong). If you prefer not to have a bath full of flowers and leaves, these could be decocted as a strong tea and strained.

AFTER SUN OIL: 0.2 ounces of rose hip oil and 0.5 ounces of Aloe Gel.

Skin Maintenance

The skin is our largest organ; it measures an average of seventeen square feet and weighs around five pounds. According to colour therapy the skin responds best to the colours green and blue (sunny country walks have always been considered to be good for the complexion).

BUTTERMILK: Cleanser for oily skin.

CIDER VINEGAR*: Diluted, as a cleanser.

COLTSFOOT: Used as a compress for thread veins.

COMFREY: As poultice to heal skin and strengthen cell formation.

HONEY: Heals cuts and wounds.

MARIGOLD tea: Used as a cleanser.

ONION: Acts as a disinfectant.

SAUERKRAUT: Used in the diet helps to heal bad skin.

SESAME OIL: Massage as a skin conditioner (with sandalwood oil for infections).

YARROW: Used as a tea for oiliness.

YOGHURT: Is a good cleanser.

*CIDER VINEGAR: As a body tone to eliminate fatigue. Restores the acid mantle of the skin. One cup in the bath for itching skin.

Aromatic Vinegars: Add half tsp of essential oil to half pint of cider vinegar (lavender or sandalwood to relax, geranium or ylang ylang to revive, etc.) or 1–8 mix of rosewater as cider vinegar as body tone.

Specific Conditions: *Folk Remedies*

SUNBURN: Yoghurt, sour cream, grated apple poultice (over the eyes), mashed cucumber, grated potato, strong tea (external), vinegar and water, vinegar and olive oil, whipped egg white with 1 tsp of honey and 1 tsp of witch hazel. All of these are useful in cooling the skin and alleviating soreness.

CORNS: Bread and butter poultice (overnight), tape on tea bags (30 mins daily), fig tree juice, milkweed.

WARTS: Crushed fresh fig on the wart (30 mins daily), used tea bag (15 mins daily for 10 days), dandelion juice (morning and evening), raw potato (bandaged overnight). Vitamin E, Aloe Vera or Chamomile Tea can be used internally to reduce lime in the system.

INSECT BITES: Eucalyptus oil (diluted) and fresh parsley—to repel. Aloe Vera and sandalwood paste can be used to heal.

BOILS: Garlic poultice, baked lemon cut in half and placed over boil, baked fig (as lemon, hold in place for 2 hours). A paste made from Ginger and turmeric powder.

WRINKLES: Apply brewers yeast and yoghurt (half in half). When dry, gently wash off with warm water and pat dry (use twice a week or alternate with a buttermilk facial—leave on for 20 mins).

FRECKLES: Rub the inside of a papaya skin over the face, leave to dry for 20 mins maximum (this treatment is very strong), will remove dead cells, tighten pores, may lighten freckles. Also try buttermilk, lemon juice, elderflower, rosewater, horseradish simmered in milk, or rosehip powder with cucumber juice. Oil or moisturize the skin after bleaching.

SAGGING FLESH: Use Vitamin E supplements both internally and externally (e.g., Evening Primrose oil, Wheat germ oil, etc.). Eat more protein, apples, sweet corn, and pulses.

DRY SKIN: External use of the following: apple juice, cider vinegar, egg yolk, melon juice, honey, liquid lecithin, and almond oil.

OILY SKIN: Parsley infusion (externally).

SCARS: Carbonised egg (cooked in frying pan without oil until black—this is best done outside, if possible, as the smell is pretty bad) use externally for several days. Vitamin E oil is good also (and easier).

RASHES: Coriander tea (internally and used as a wash).

Herbal Skincare

The skin is our most exposed organ; both internal toxins and environmental pollutants affect it. Useful herbs for the care of the skin will include cleansing herbs such as Echinacea, yellow dock, and burdock; silica bearing herbs such as stinging nettle, yucca, and horsetail; and (because many skin disorders can be aggravated by stress) relaxing herbs such as passiflora and Californian Poppy.

ACNE: Is usually associated with puberty and can be helped by eating more selectively: avoiding the use of nuts (especially peanut butter), fried foods, shell fish, animal fats, cheese, sugar, chocolate, colas, coffee, alcohol.

Aloe Vera juice can be taken internally and a paste of turmeric and sandalwood used externally, cucumber juice and watercress leaves can be used as a poultice.

HERPES: Known in China to be a "damp heat" condition, characterized by wet, pus filled blisters (often in the genital region). Although herpes is contagious, there is some evidence to show that it is more likely to be contracted by people with an imbalance of the amino acids arginine and lysine. Supplements of lysine and reduction of arginine bearing foods (including nuts, seeds, chocolate, oats, wheat, etc.) can help to remedy this imbalance.

Red clover tea can help to detoxify the body, and a poultice of bentonite clay allowed to dry, then removed and replaced with a salve of golden seal and myrrh on the affected area will reduce blistering and itchiness.

ECZEMA: affects at least five percent of the population. Its symptoms include inflammation, dryness, and blisters (most common on the knees and elbows).

The causes of eczema include: nutritional deficiency, allergies, stress, and a weakened immune system.

Dairy is the most common allergy and eczema is the most common symptom.

To treat eczema it is advisable to avoid milk products, wheat (if an allergy occurs), alcohol, sugar, and nicotine. The diet should include fish oils as they contain EPA (rich in Vitamin A that reduces inflammation). Echinacea is an herb, which has strong anti-inflammatory properties; it will also speed healing and stimulate the immune system.

The formula **Yellow Dock Skin Cleanse** can be effective in treating the above three conditions (Acne, Herpes, and Eczema), this formula contains many of the above-mentioned herbs.

PSORIASIS: affects three percent of the population and is generally considered to be incurable (so let's say it may require a bit more time and energy). The causes of psoriasis include: poor digestion of protein, excessive alcohol consumption, lack of sunlight, excessive manufacture of skin cells (caused by faulty liver function), or shortage of hydrochloric acid in the stomach.

Useful supplements in the treatment of psoriasis include: G.L.A. (evening primrose, borage, and blackcurrant seeds provide good sources of this nutrient) Vitamin A, zinc, Vitamin C, selenium, and Vitamin B complex. The herb Milk Thistle contains large quantities of silymarin, which protects the liver (silymarin has even been used successfully to prevent death from death cap mushroom). Sarsaparilla is also good for the liver and found to have beneficial effects on psoriasis; it can be taken as a tea for all skin problems.

The formula **Bupleurum Liver Cleanse** contains sylmarin, bupleurum, Oregon grape, and dandelion—all very effective in improving liver function. The latter formula can be combined with **Yellow Dock Skin Cleanse** in treating psoriasis.[3]

Skin problems often express much of what is happening within the body. Modern treatments (such as steroid creams, etc.) suppress the body's natural signals and give us the impression that the disorder has been dealt with. If, however, we do not treat the underlying cause, that imbalance will continue to express itself in different and more pronounced ways, until we get the message.

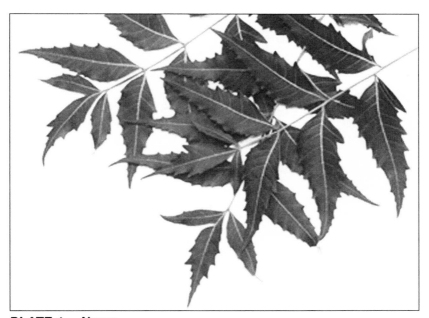

PLATE 1. Neem.

Key Herb for the Skin: Neem *(Azadarishta Indica)*

Neem is considered to be a principle plant in Ayurvedic medicine, and as a result the Neem tree is encouraged to grow throughout India. Its leaves are used to treat skin problems, its twigs are used as toothbrushes, and its bark, seeds, and oil are rich in more than thirty biologically active ingredients.

PROPERTIES: anti-inflammatory, insecticidal, anti-septic, anti-fungal, analgesic.

Neem is found to be effective against various bacteria (including staphylococcus aureus) and seen to have a comparable effect to cortisone in treating skin conditions such as eczema.

Neem extracts are now commonly used in anti-dandruff shampoos, skin treatment creams, salves, and lotions or taken internally in tablet or capsule form. Neem seed oil is commercially used as a natural insecticide.

CHAPTER THREE

Wild & Free

I REMEMBER, BACK IN THE early seventies, having a very knowledgeable lodger who took my partner and me on a foraging expedition just a few miles out of town. The result was sufficient wild food to supplement our diet for at least a week.

On a Himalayan trek in the eighties, what would otherwise have been a six week period of lentils, potatoes, and onions was made more interesting and nutritious for my wife and me, by supplementing our diet with such foods as wild spinach (fat hen), young fern tops, wild herbs, and wild fruits.

Those of us who live in the city, where concrete and pollutants often dominate our awareness, tend to overlook that we still have a lot of fairly unspoiled countryside and hedgerows where wild food can be found in abundance.

Before we start our foraging, however, we need to remember that since 1975 it has been illegal (for sound ecological reasons) to uproot wild plants without obtaining the permission of the owner of the land on which they grow. With the more endangered species, it is forbidden also to take the flowers or seeds. Many of the more common wild plants are edible; so if we are selective and only take a few leaves or stalks from each plant, we need not damage the environment in order to get a few food supplements. If we want to use the roots of wild plants, it is now possible to buy seeds of burdock, comfrey, horseradish, etc., so that we can grow our own and preserve the balance of nature. We are familiar with obvious hedgerow foods such as hazelnuts and blackberries, but overlook acorns (a good coffee substitute), pine nuts, and beech masts.

BURDOCK: (known in Somerset as "wild rhubarb") The stems of this plant, peeled and sliced, are delicious cooked in butter. In Japan the root is used as a vegetable or boiled as tea; it has a strong flavour and quality.

COMFREY LEAVES: Are delicious (when young) fried in batter as tempura.

DANDELION LEAVES: Are good as a salad or green vegetable. The flowers make a good wine, and the roots make a good (bitter tasting) root vegetable or (roasted and ground) are ideal as a coffee substitute.

ELDERBERRIES: Cooked with crab apples, provide a sweet/sour flavor.

FAT HEN: (Wild Spinach) contains more B1, calcium, iron, and protein than cabbage.

GREEN VEGETABLES: Why not try ground elder, the young leaves of red valerian, stinging nettle, chickweed, or shepherd's purse? All of these can be cooked with butter, wild garlic (or spring onions), and a dash of lemon juice.

HORSERADISH JUICE: is a powerful expectorant for respiratory congestion.

NETTLES: Make a good soup, beer, or tea.

ROSE HIPS: Contain twenty times the Vitamin C of oranges—first remove hairy seeds and prepare as syrups or jams.

ROSE PETALS: Can be added to various dishes. They are high in Vitamin C and Quercetin, cooling and calming to the spirit.

SALADS: Can be enhanced by the addition of wild herbs such as marjoram, mint, and thyme. For a change try finely sliced burdock stems, sorrel leaves, or the purple petals of lesser knapweed.

SLOES: Can be pickled in salt (as with olives or umeboshi plum).

SORREL: Can also be used for making a delicate lemon-flavoured sauce, perfect for fish dishes, but the juice of wild sorrel can be mildly toxic if used to excess.

WILD TEAS: Can be made from lime flowers, the dried flower heads of heather and many other herbs.

Fungi

There are, of course, hundreds of edible fungi; few of them are used due to the danger of incorrect identification—many toadstools are extremely poisonous.

CHANTERELLES: Cannot be easily confused with any dangerous fungi; they are excellent fried with eggs and aromatic herbs.

GIANT PUFFBALLS: Are delicious sliced and fried as steaks.

BEEFSTEAK FUNGUS: Has a slightly acrid flavour, which can be improved on with the addition of sweet herbs.

BLEWITTS: Require a little extra cooking but have a very rich flavour. They are often found in "fairy rings." The Wood Blewitt is bluish or violet when young, turning reddish with age.

Warning: When gathering fungi or any other wild food, be sure you have a good understanding of what not to eat—if in doubt leave it out—mistakes are often fatal.

Also, be wary of picking wild foods from areas which may be subject to pesticide sprays, or too close to main roads and therefore prone to high levels of lead, cadmium, and other toxins. I would also avoid anything growing near pylons, phone masts, and electricity generating stations (the list is, unfortunately, becoming endless).

Who knows, in this time of economic downturn some of the above information may prove useful in providing variety and free nutrition to an otherwise compromised diet.

Flowers as Medicine

"There is enough beauty, truth and nourishment in one small flower to last a lifetime"
—Amancio D'Silva

CHAMOMILE: Flowers and hops can be used as a poultice for pain. Chamomile tea is not only a mild sedative, but also rich in calcium.

CHRYSANTHEMUM: Flowers cooked down, as strong tea will help to rid the body of worms. Chrysanthemum tea can be taken to relieve headaches, reduce fevers, and hypertension or used as a mild wash for inflammatory disorders of the eye.

GOLDEN ROD: Flowers are useful as a diuretic tea and a wash for psoriasis.

HONEYSUCKLE: Flowers can be used as a tea for both flu and arthritis.

MARIGOLD: (calendula) Flowers make a good poultice for bruising. Marigold tea can be used for cleansing the skin or taken to relieve pre-menstrual syndrome.

MULLEIN: The flowers of Mullein (verbascum) have strong nervine and analgesic properties.

RED CLOVER: The flowers of red clover can be cooked down as a tarry paste to treat skin cancers. The flowers can also be used as a tea; they are high in phyto-estrogens and cleansing for the blood.

ROSES: Rose Petals, Cornflowers, and Chamomile flowers boiled together for a few minutes and used between muslin (when cooled) as compresses improve brightness of the eyes.

The Rose was one of the major medicines used in mediaeval Europe, Asia, and Arabia.

VIOLET: Flowers as tea (sweetened with honey) for nervous tension.

Foods as "Barefoot Doctor" Medicines

> *"The Cabbage leaf is the Doctor of the Poor"*
> —Dr. Blanc 1881

EXTERNAL USE

CABBAGE: Sauerkraut poultice is good for stomach-aches and rheumatism. Cabbage and olive oil poultice for breast lumps.

CUCUMBER: Mashed with grated potato for sunburn.

DAIKON (Mooli Radish) or TURNIP Plasters: Grate the Daikon or Turnip add a little white flour to make a sticky mess, wrap in muslin, and apply to areas of heat, pain, bruising, or over areas relating to internal bleeding.

DAIKON: Juice is also good for bruising, headaches, bites, and burns.

TOFU Plaster: Mash tofu with a little white flour and a small amount of grated ginger; apply to skin to absorb fever and reduce swelling.

FIG TREE Juice or MILKWEED Juice: Applied to corns and calluses.

GINGER BATH: To improve circulation and to help in cases of dysentery. Grate four or five ounces of fresh root ginger into a muslin sack, attach sack to hot water tap, and let hot water run through. Then squeeze out into bathwater.

MISO: Use as a plaster (on cheesecloth). Used for bleeding, itching skin, or swellings.

MUSTARD BATH: As a footbath for cold, etc., or whole bath as stimulant recirculation, etc. CAUTION: Mustard will burn, so use as appropriate for your skin's sensitivity.

POTATO: Juice for rheumatism.

SALT: Is extremely "Yang" and can therefore be used to help counteract "Yin" toxins.

"Yin" toxins include all poisons, most drugs, and radiation.

Hot Salt packs are useful in cases of abdominal and menstrual cramps, muscle stiffness, and to calm diarrhoea. Care should be taken to ensure the pack is not too hot. Cloth can be used between the skin and the salt pack, and then it should be removed as pack cools.

YOGHURT: Useful in the relief of sunburn.

INTERNAL USE

LEEKS: Are good vegetables in cases of high blood pressure.

LETTUCE: Can help to combat insomnia. (Wild Lettuce is a potent sedative.)

SPINACH: Is good for digestion, liver issues, kidney stones, and rheumatism.

WATERCRESS: Is high in iodine and many other trace elements. It is useful for people who are overweight.

THE ONION: Can be used as a poultice for pain and ear infections and boils (cooked for latter). Onion juice can be taken with honey for colds or used to treat itching from bee stings (once the sting has been removed).

The onion is a symbol of immortality; its many layers represent the removal of veils of ignorance. To dream of an onion is good luck. It is an emblem of deity with the Druids and ancient Egyptians, and it was used for divining purposes in early England.

As regards medicine, the onion contains sulphur, acts as a diuretic, stimulant, and expectorant. It is a recommended cure for deafness (the juice dropped into the ear, diluted with warm olive oil). The juice can also be used for chilblains, burns, insect bites, and stings, or taken with honey for asthma.

From a dietary viewpoint, in macrobiotics the onion is considered "Yin" (acidic) but acceptable as food, whereas in the Indian Brahman culture it is often prohibited due to its "rajasic" (stimulating, aphrodisiac) nature.

Food Antidotes *(not intended for allergies, merely excesses)*

FOOD ANTIDOTES

CHEESE and DAIRY: Black Pepper or Cayenne.

SUGARS: Dry ginger powder.

EGGS: Turmeric.

TOBACCO: Gotu kola, calamus root, celery seeds.

RED MEAT: Cayenne, cloves.

PEANUT BUTTER: Ginger.

ALCOHOL: Cumin or coriander seeds.

TEA: Ginger.

CAFFEINE and Chocolate: Nutmeg with cardamom.

The above antidotes should ideally be used with the food concerned; e.g., one or two cardamom seeds ground with the coffee beans, a small pinch of ginger in the tea, scrambled eggs cooked with a pinch of turmeric, etc.

CHAPTER FOUR

Food & Health

"He who takes medicine and neglects diet wastes the skills of the physician."
—Chinese Proverb

"Instead of eating well, getting enough sleep, and stopping our constant criticism of ourselves, our busy, scattered, rushed lives force us to do the opposite. And our incomplete self screams for the attention of that which is lost."
—Carlos Castaneda

"Pay heed to the providing of nourishment and what a man seeks to fill his own mouth with."
—I Ching *(Chinese Book of Changes)*

"Eating is a sacred alchemy."
—Taisha Abelar

First the Bad News

1. Food related deaths exceed those caused by car accidents; these include factors such as obesity, diabetes, colon cancer and food toxicity.

2. Obesity (due largely to inappropriate eating) is responsible for 325,000 deaths annually.
3. Most people are currently estimated to have 300–500 chemicals in their bodies, which have been introduced in the food chain in the last fifty years.
4. Between ten and thirty percent of adolescent girls are iron deficient.[4]
5. The average American consumes the equivalent of 28 tsp of sugar daily.
6. The average European is now 10 kg heavier than twenty years ago.
7. It takes an estimated ecological footprint of 24 acres of land to sustain an American (Britain is catching up rapidly)—whereas to sustain an Indian takes less than 1 acre.
8. Microwaves change the structure of food; they have been banned in Russia since 1976 due to the formation of carcinogens in microwave cooked meat, dairy, fruit, and vegetables.
9. There are 500,000 pesticide related poisonings per year, worldwide.

The above points are just a few of the reasons why it is important that we are conscious about what we eat, and from where we source our food. In the modern world there are so many dietary approaches. Some are good; others can be disastrous in the long term. It is probably more useful to look at diets that have stood the test of time—the traditional diets of each culture.

So what is a traditional diet?

Many people would automatically assume that the traditional British diet was made up of Roast beef and potatoes, or fish and chips, but we have to remember that going back in history meat and fish would have only been available to wealthy landowners. The majority of the population would have only eaten these foods if they could poach them from the landlord (or if they lived near the sea—in the case of fish).

Potatoes were only introduced in the sixteenth century (along with tomatoes, aubergine, tobacco, and other members of the nightshade family). Up until that time the average person would have lived on grains, such as barley, etc. (rice was also grown in the fens before they were drained); vegetables; fruits (in season); nuts (in season); and wild foods, such as fungi, chickweed, dandelion, berries, etc. So the traditional British diet would be quite similar to that in China, India, Japan, and other ancient cultures.

Many nutritionists consider the Korean diet to be the best approach to balanced eating. It is made up of seventy percent carbohydrates (including rice and vegetables), seventeen percent protein (including meats, fish, tofu, and pulses), and very low in fat. The average Western Diet is approx forty percent carbohydrates, fifteen to twenty percent fats, fifteen to twenty percent sugars, and generally higher in protein.

Obviously diets may need to vary according to climate, etc. The Eskimo will need much higher levels of fat and protein, whereas someone in Southern California may do quite well on salads, fruits, nuts, and seeds (but neither of these approaches would be of long term benefit to those living in Northern Europe). Although we import vast quantities of tropical fruits, etc., these are not necessarily good for us on a regular basis and definitely not good for the environment in terms of the carbon footprint.

FRUIT: The fruits that have least calories include the berries (such as blueberries, cranberry, loganberry, gooseberry, and blackberry). These are all very nutritious and high in vitamins and other protective nutrients (such as bio-flavinoids, etc.)—4 oz (100gm) of these fruits will contain an average of 15 calories, and they grow easily in Northern Europe and North America. Whereas the sweeter or richer fruits such as figs, dates, and avocado will be richer in calories 2–300 calories per 100 gm. And they generally require major transportation. Fruits should be eaten, ideally, during their season. Excessive use of fruit in cooler, damper climates is not advised, due to their cooling nature and their proximity to sugars. Dried fruits travel well and are high in nutrients, just a few blueberries, wolfberries, or dates will provide a great deal of nourishment.

The only traditionally vegetarian culture is India, for several reasons:

1. The cow is sacred, so its products (such as milk, ghee, etc., are precious foods and therefore not polluted with hormonal and antibiotic drugs)—milk is never taken cold, but scalded (twice) before drinking.
2. Food is usually well cooked.
3. The major focus regarding diet and health in India is "AGNI" (digestive fire), so spices are a necessary aid in improving digestion and destroying "AMA"(undigested foods).

Digestive Spices Include: Cinnamon, Ginger, Pepper, Cayenne, Fennel seed, Turmeric, Cumin, Cardamom, Coriander (some of these should be used with care by people with a fiery constitution).

CHAPTER FIVE

·

The Five Elements, Food, Herbs, Health & Healing

IN TRADITIONAL DIETS THE INCLUSION of the elements are of particular importance; certain foods support certain elements and the organ systems related to those elements. I feel that this is a better way of approaching diet than getting too caught up with nutrition.

Nutrition is important of course, but keeping the system energetically balanced is more liable to lead to good health than resorting to supplements or eating foods that are high in a particular nutrient, regardless of whether that food is suited to our constitution.

The Chinese base many of their healing systems (acupuncture, feng shui, herbal medicine, etc.) on **Five Element Theory**—a system used in China for hundreds, if not thousands of years, and considered to be the basis of man's relationship to the natural environment.

THE FIRE ELEMENT

ORGAN: Relates to the heart.

SEASON: Summer.

TIME: 11 a.m.–3 p.m.

COLOUR: Red.

EMOTION: Anxiety.

VIRTUE: Joy.

SOUND: Laughter.

SMELL: Scorched.

TASTE: Bitter.

BEST FOODS: Include leaves, flowers.

COOKING STYLE: Dry roasting.

FLOWERS: Rose Petals and Elderflowers.

HERBS: Aloe, Chaparral, Roasted Dandelion Root, Hawthorn, Zizyphus seed.

NEEDS: To Drain, cool, and calm

KEY WORDS: Inner Vision—The Heart is the home of Shen.[5]

THE EARTH ELEMENT

ORGAN: Relates to the spleen, an important organ in digestion and assimilation.

SEASON: Late Summer.

TIME: 7–11 a.m.

COLOUR: Yellow.

EMOTION: Pensiveness.

VIRTUE: Equanimity.

SOUND: Song.

SMELL: Fragrant.

TASTE: Sweet

FOODS: To include yellow and orange grains and root vegetables, medicinal mushrooms, ripened gooseberries, blackberries and rosehips, and mild digestive spices.

COOKING STYLE: Steamed food is best.

HERBS: Ginseng, Astragalus, Codonopsis, Atractylodes, and Licorice.

NEEDS: To tonify, to harmonize.

John E. Smith

KEY WORDS: Acquired Qi—Purpose, Intent.

THE METAL ELEMENT

ORGAN: Relates to the lung.

SEASON: Autumn.

TIME: 3–7 a.m.

COLOUR: White, Silver.

EMOTION: Grief.

VIRTUE: Courage.

SOUND: Sob.

SMELL: Rotten.

TASTE: Pungent, Spicy.

FOODS: Responds well to baked foods (particularly the onion family) plus seeds, nuts, horseradish, and dandelion root (not roasted—as roasting relates to fire element).

COOKING STYLE: Baked.

HERBS: Comfrey Root, Mullein, Fritillary, and Loquat.

NEEDS: To disperse.

KEYWORDS: "Wei Qi"—Protection. Corporeal Soul, The Seven "Po."[6]

THE WATER ELEMENT

ORGANS: Relates to the kidneys and bladder.

SEASON: Winter.

TIME: 3–7 p.m.

COLOUR: Blue, Black.

EMOTION: Fear, Fright.

VIRTUE: Wisdom.

SOUND: Groan.

SMELL: Putrid.

TASTE: Salt.

FOODS: The best foods would be sprouted grains (particularly barley and seeds [seed energy])—sea foods and chickweed are also good.

COOKING STYLE: Boiling.

HERBS: Parsley, Rehmania.

NEEDS: To purge, soften.

KEYWORDS: "Jing" (Essence). "Zhi" (Will).

THE WOOD ELEMENT:

ORGAN: Relates to the liver.

SEASON: Spring.

TIME: 11 p.m.–3 a.m.

COLOUR: Green.

EMOTION: Anger.

VIRTUE: Kindness.

SOUND: Shout.

TASTE: Sour.

COOKING METHOD: Sauté.

FOODS: Lightly sautéed stems and leaves are good and dandelion leaves. Orange peel, rosehips, and sloes are all excellent for the liver.

HERBS: Peony, Bupleurum.

NEEDS: Toning and Consolidation.

KEYWORDS: Outer Vision. The 3 'Hun."[7]

Food Therapy

THE FIVE FLAVOURS: *Using Foods to Suit the Body's Needs.*

SALT: Moistens, Softens, Holds Water, Detoxifies.

EXAMPLES: Sea Vegetables.
ORGANS: Kidney/Bladder.

SOUR: Gathers—Astringent (good for "leaking" or "sagging").
EXAMPLES: Lemon, Schizandra.
ORGANS: Lung/Large Intestine.

BITTER: Drains, Dries, Improves Appetite and Digestion.
EXAMPLES: Dandelion, Dark Greens.
ORGANS: Heart / Small Intestine.

SWEET: Harmonizes.
Two types of Sweetness (Full and Empty). Full Nourishes and Empty fools the body and weakens Spleen.
EXAMPLES: Full = meats, rice, starchy roots. Empty = fruits, sugars.
ORGANS: Spleen/Stomach/Pancreas.

PUNGENT: Disperses Stagnation.
EXAMPLES: Garlic, Asafoetida, and Fenugreek.
ORGANS: Liver/Gall Bladder.

FOODS, WHICH DRIVE OUT COLD: Acerola Cherry, Ginger, Onion Family, Malt, Peach, Turnip. Sweet Potato, Wines, Chestnut, Black Pepper, Anchovy, Pine Kernels, Mussels, Trout, Sweet Rice, Nutmeg, Spearmint, Mustard Leaf, Longan, Squash, Cayenne, Walnut, Chicken, Lambs Kidney.
SPECIFIC HERBS: Cinnamon (Rou Gui).

FOODS WHICH CLEAR HEAT: (True heat as opposed to "false heat" which is treated as Yin deficiency)—Asparagus, Banana, Elderflower, Mung, Millet, Grapefruit, Tofu, Peppermint, Clam, Potato, and Watermelon.
SPECIFIC HERBS: Rehmania (Sheng Di Huang), Dandelion, Chrysanthemum.

FOODS TO NOURISH BLOOD: (Blood deficien\cy, anaemia, Insomnia, Feeling undernourished, Out of touch, Spaced out, Disturbed shen.)—Leafy Greens, Aduki, Beetroot, Watercress, Sweet Rice, Apricots, Figs, Nettle, and Dandelion.

SPECIFIC HERBS: Chinese Angelica (Dang Gui), Polyganum (He Shou Wu).

COOKING METHODS & THEIR EFFECTS ON FOODS:

RAW FOODS: Cooling.

STEAMED: Cooling to Neutral.

BOILED: Neutral. STEWED: Neutral.

STIR FRY: Warming.

BAKED: More Warming.

ROASTED: Heating. GRILLED: More Heating.

BARBECUED: Most Heating.

CHAPTER SIX

Getting to the Heart of the Matter

BECAUSE SO MUCH IS KNOWN about the causes of heart problems, they could potentially be the easiest of all conditions to prevent or even cure. Reliance on coronary bi-pass operations, nitro-glycerine, and other powerful drug therapies has left us, however, with heart conditions reaching epidemic proportions, killing more people per year than all cancers combined. Isn't it time we started making some connections, and stopped viewing the heart (and other organ systems) as being isolated from the rest of the body?

Diet, exercise, stress management, and herbal therapies are all valid ways of maintaining a healthy heart. It may often have been one of these approaches that has kept many people off of the operating table and away from potentially dangerous drugs.

DIET: The major focus of the diet needs to revolve around the use of complex carbohydrates, in the form of whole grains (rice, oats, etc.); freshly cooked vegetables; and smaller amounts of beans, pulses, fruits, meat, and dairy products.

FOODS TO AVOID:

Fats: A build up of fats in the arteries is the main cause of heart disease. This leads to arterial occlusion, thrombosis, and subsequent heart attack.

Sugars: Excessive consumption of sugars may be a greater contributing factor to the build up of cholesterol than the consumption of cholesterol itself.

Excessive use: Of red meats, white flour products, and salt.

Western and Eastern natural practitioners use many different herbs to treat conditions of the heart. There has been extensive research into the effects of Tienchi Ginseng (a cardio tonic used in China to treat gunshot and stab wounds). Tienchi acts to dissolve blood clots, lower cholesterol, promote circulation, and reduce trauma. The mild relaxant Dong Quai (Chinese Angelica) actually prevents the build up of arterial plaque. Hawthorn Berry regulates the heart rate, controls hypertension, and has been found to reduce the incidence of angina pectoris. Hawthorn berries contain flavinoids, which have a strengthening effect on the cell walls of the heart. The Latin name for Motherwort (Leonoris cardiaca) refers to its beneficial action on the heart. Motherwort not only lowers blood pressure, but is also an effective diuretic (diuretics are still the most commonly prescribed drugs for hypertension.)

Useful Food Herbs

HAWTHORN BERRIES:

Ruler: Mars.

Tissues: Plasma, blood, and muscles.

Actions: Stimulant, carminative, vasodilator, diuretic.

Indications: Weak heart, hypertension, palpitations, insomnia, food stagnation, and abdominal tension.

Hawthorn berries strengthen the heart muscles and reduce cholesterol, promoting longevity.

CRANBERRY JUICE: Could reduce the risk of heart disease by forty percent (by reducing cholesterol).[8]

ROSE: Opens the mind and heart.

The rose is known in the Middle East as "The flower of devotional worship" and "the lotus of the heart."

SUPPLEMENTS:

Vitamin E Prevents abnormal blood clotting.

Vitamin F Lowers blood cholesterol.

CoQ10: (ubiquinone, Vitamin Q) CoQ10 is a naturally occurring compound, which plays a key role in energy production. Those suffering from heart failure are generally found to possess lower levels of this valuable nutrient, as are those using certain pharmaceutical drugs aimed at treating heart conditions, including some beta blockers and statins

We are all ultimately responsible for our own health. It is therefore our responsibility to learn as much as we can to help ourselves, so that surgery and drug therapy are the exception rather than the rule.

Other herbs of relevance include Longan, Chinese Ziziphus, Passiflora, Valerian, Chamomile, and many Ayurvedic "Medya Rasayana" herbs (Bacopa, Hydrocotyl Asiatica, Ashwagandha, Tulsi, and Sarpagandha).

Herbs for the Heart and Nervous System

1) CHINESE ZIZYPHUS SEED (*Zizyphus jujube.*)

Zizyphus is usually referred to as the seed of a wild date (jujube) from the family of buckthorn. It is lentil-like in appearance, can be eaten (best combined with berries such as lycium), or added to decoctions. Its flavour is sweet/sour.

Actions: Nourishes heart and stabilizes spirit (shen).

Uses: Anxiety, irritability, insomnia, and palpitations. Suan zao ren also acts as an oxygenator (re altitude sickness), and its regular use can brighten the complexion.

Properties: Nutritive, nervine, sedative, analgesic, high in saponins.

Zizyphus is a major ingredient in many traditional Chinese herbal formulae including Gui Pi Tang.

2) LONGAN (*Euphoria longan, dimocarpus longan, long yan rou,* "dragon's eye.")

Longan is a Chinese fruit similar to lychee but with a smoother shell. It is valued in China as a major blood tonic, useful in strengthening both heart and spleen, and it is described as a "Shen" (spirit) herb.

Active Ingredients: Vitamin A, Vitamin C, protein, and Iron (Longan contains approximately fifteen times the iron as that found in spinach).

Uses: Longan can be useful in cases of anaemia, insomnia, amnesia, dizziness, and low stamina.

Longan can be used as a food or medicine.

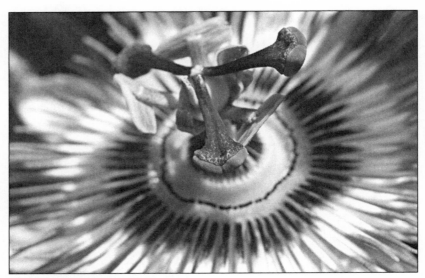

PLATE 2.   Passionflower.

3) PASSIFLORA (passion flower, *passiflora incarnata, grenadilla*, "wild apricot vine," "maypop.")

There is a great deal of evidence to indicate native people grew passiflora for food and medicine centuries before the Europeans arrived in the Americas.

This beautiful plant was first brought to Europe from Brazil in the seventeenth century and is said to represent the passion of Christ.

Uses: Passiflora is useful in cases of hysteria, epilepsy, attention deficit disorder, extreme anxiety, insomnia, diarrhoea, and dysentery. It combines well with valerian, Chinese loquat, rosa damascene, and hawthorn.

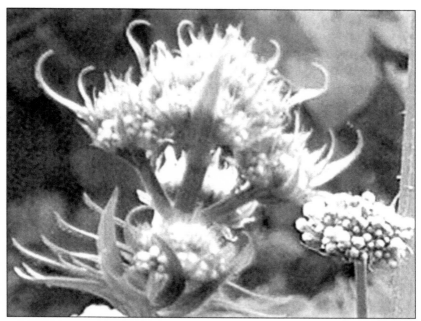

PLATE 3.   Valerian Flower.

4) VALERIAN (*v. officinalis*, "all heal.")

Valerian has been used medicinally since the time of Hippocrates and Galen as an aromatic and diuretic herb. Generally classified as a warming sedative and nervine tonic, it became known in the sixteenth century as a cure for epilepsy. In the Second World War valerian was widely used in the treatment of PCS ("shell shock"). The name of the plant is attributed to the Latin word *valere* meaning "to be in good health."

The whole plant has a foetid smell, which can be attractive to cats (the French name for valerian is "herbe aux chats"). I well remember a local Tomcat who was known to leap several feet in the air in order to reach valerian roots hanging to dry from my clothesline. The active compound *actnidine* mimics the smell of cat urine. Rats are also attracted to the smell of valerian (rats infected with a certain parasite are actually attracted to the smell of cat urine[9]). It is said that the Pied Piper of Hamlyn owed his success to copious amounts of valerian concealed in his clothing.

Eastern valerian (*tagar, v. wallichii*) and related plants such as jatamansi and spikenard were traditionally used as perfumes, incense, and anointing oils due to their higher concentration of aromatic oils. In America the increasingly endangered Ladies Slipper orchid is often given the name "American valerian" due to its similar properties.

N.B. Valerian officinalis should not be confused with the garden variety (Centranthus), which can be used as a vegetable, but does not possess pronounced medicinal properties.

5) SARPAGANDHA: (*rauwolfia serpentina*, "Indian snakeroot," "insanity herb," "moonshine plant.")

History: Known since the time of Caraka (first century A.D) as a potent sedative.

It is said that Mahatma Gandhi chewed the root to attain a state of detachment during meditation.

Actions: Sedative, antihypertensive, neuroleptic, and hypnotic.

Uses: To treat high blood pressure. In the 1940s it was used successfully to treat one million Indian people with high blood pressure. The name "Indian Snakeroot" refers to its use both internally and topically in the treatment of snakebite.

Active Ingredients: The main active ingredient "*reserpine*" became famous in the 1950s when it was used as an alternative to lobotomy and electric shock therapy for treating certain types of mental illness.[10] Reserpine had become known in 1934 as the world's first anti-hypertensive drug (Serpina), after it was discovered that Burmese elephants were given Sarpagandha root to calm them.

In Alchemy: Sarpagandha relates to "animal energy," the wolf and the snake (rauwolfia serpentina). It is said to help in the avoidance of "double danger." (This is seen with "bi-polar" patients, where depression will alternate with levels of high excitation.) Sarpagandha also helps those with a fear of snakes or dogs, or who dream repeatedly of snakes and wolves. Sarpagandha also relates to the DNA helix and the "cosmic snake" or *kundalini*.[11]

6) CHAMOMILE: (*Matricaria recutita*)

Known in the United States as "Band Aid for the Stomach" and used for many disorders affecting both the nervous and digestive systems and in the case of menstrual cramps. Chamomile's easily assimilated calcium content makes it excellent for children in assisting the development of teeth and bones, whilst treating colic and irritability caused by teething.

Active Constituents: Volatile oils, anthelmic acid, flavinoids, tannin.

Properties: Nervine, carminative, sedative, antiseptic, emmenagogue.

Chamomile contains a high concentration of easily assimilable calcium (a mild sedative), which makes this herb useful in soothing the nerves, muscles, and digestive system. Chamomile can also be useful in helping to alleviate menstrual cramps. Applied externally in creams or lotions, chamomile can be used in the treatment of rashes, soreness, and joint pain.

Key Formula: Gui Pi Tang

First recorded: Thirteenth century A.D. ("Formulas to Aid the Living")

Actions: Although Gui Pi Tang is used primarily to "Tonify Spleen Qi and Nourish Heart Blood," it is considered to be a formula that treats several disorders with the same method. This formula addresses two main organ functions, which in turn affect the entire system. First Gui Pi Tang warms the spleen thereby improving digestion and the transformation of food into blood and energy, this naturally improves heart blood and as a result calms and nourishes the spirit of the heart (shen).

The main emotion of the spleen is worry (or pensiveness) and the heart, of course, is adversely affected by excessive worry or over-thinking, this formula will benefit both of these major organ systems.

Uses: Anxiety, dream disturbed sleep, insomnia, night sweats, palpitations, fatigue, amnesia.

Gui Pi Tang contains many energy tonic herbs including Ginseng and Astragalus (both major herbs for the spleen and lung) together with the blood tonics Chinese Angelica and Longan. These herbs are enhanced by Red Date fruit and seed (Zizyphus), Poria fungus, and Polygala Root; the latter three herbs all strengthen the heart and calm the spirit.

CHAPTER SEVEN

"Venting the Spleen"

THE SPLEEN IS THE ORGAN of adaptation, nourishment, and support, the organ of transformation and transportation. The spleen is a central organ in Chinese Medicine. The term "spleen" often applies to the whole of the "middle jiao," (which includes stomach, intestines, pancreas, and part of the liver).

The physical expression of the spleen is digestion, but there is a mental side to its function: we don't only digest food but also digest knowledge and information; we don't only eat for nutrition but also for comfort.

The spleen is the "mother organ" it provides support and nourishment; its element is earth. Being "grounded" or "at home" in our body is an expression of good spleen energy or "Qi."

> *"The stomach and spleen are a yin/yang pivot, they transform the substances that are 'not you' to the substances that are you."*
>
> —Dr. Michael Tierra

Major Approaches to Nourishing the Spleen:

1. Eat a balanced diet avoiding too many cold, wet, and refined foods.
2. Chew well! "The stomach has no teeth."
3. Avoid excessive mental work or worry.

MAJOR SPLEEN PROBLEM: Qi Deficiency and Dampness.

The sweet flavour belongs to the earth element; the spleen therefore responds well to "Full" sweet foods, which include meats, rice, and starchy roots. "Empty" sweet foods, fruits, sugars, etc., convert to gas and water; they fool the body and weaken spleen function.

FOODS TO ENLIVEN SPLEEN QI:

Energetic Fish: Herring, Mackerel, Eel, Octopus, etc.

Most meat: Beef, Chicken, and Rabbit.

Pulses: Lentils, Tofu (well cooked and well seasoned).

Sweet Vegetables: Sweet potatoes, Squash, Carrots, etc.

Grains: Rice, etc.

Nourishing Fruits: Dates, Figs, Longan, etc.

Sweeter Root Herbs: Ginseng, Astragalus, Liquorice, etc.

Herbs for the Spleen

N.B. Two of the key herbs for the spleen are Panax Ginseng and Astragalus, these are both included above. For further details of these major herbs, see my earlier book 100 Herbs of Power.

1) CODONOPSIS ROOT (*dang shen*)

Codonopsis is an adaptogenic[12] herb, rather like ginseng in its action, only milder and often more appropriate for long-term treatment. Its energy is neutral, its flavour is sweet, and it is used as a tonic for both spleen and lungs. In Chinese Medicine, formulas normally requiring ginseng may use Codonopsis as a substitute, as it is cheaper, more plentiful, and has similar properties; for this to be acceptable a much larger amount of Codonopsis is required (three to four times the amount of ginseng recommended for the formula). Often smaller amounts of ginseng will be used, accompanied by larger amounts of Codonopsis.

Uses: Codonopsis can be used as a general tonic, in cases of anaemia, asthma and lung weakness, cancer, diarrhoea, poor digestion, prolapse (including haemorrhoids), and to increase breast milk with nursing mothers.

There are no reported side effects with even long-term usage of Codonopsis. In China pieces of Codonopsis root are given to babies for the purpose of teething.

2) PSEUDOSTELLARIA *(tai zi shen)*

Pseudostellaria is a neutral, sweet, slightly bitter, Qi tonic for the lungs and spleen; it is similar to codonopsis but more active in promoting body fluids. It has stronger Qi properties than American Ginseng, is excellent for fatigue, weak digestion, shortness of breath, and a good herb for use in advanced stages of degenerative diseases.

Key Formula for Spleen Qi Deficiency— Bu Zhong Yi Qi Tang

(**Ginseng & Astragalus Formula**—"Tonify the Centre to Invigorate Qi Pills")

This is a primary strengthening herbal compound used by traditional herbalists throughout the Orient. This formula is designed to pick up "sagging qi" (including such symptoms as low energy, poor digestion, diarrhoea, and prolapse) and is useful for long-term deficiency syndrome such as malnutrition and wasting disorders.

Traditional Uses: Bu Zhong Yi Qi Wan is a classical formula for tonifying stomach and spleen qi, invigorating liver qi, and raising yang. It was originally used to treat prolapse of organs (including prolapse of rectum, uterus, and colon and such conditions as varicose veins, haemorrhoids, and hernia). This formula is also useful for uterine bleeding and habitual miscarriage.

Ingredients: Ginseng (ren shen), Astragalus, Liquorice, Chinese angelica, Cimicifuga, Codonopsis, Atractylodes, Citrus peel, Bupleurum, Jujube dates, and Ginger root.

On a Clear Day You Can Smell the Candida

MEANINGFUL DIAGNOSTICS VERSUS "THE DUSTBIN" OF MODERN MEDICINE

My mention of Candida brings to light a classic example of the "dustbin" diagnostics of modern western medicine. I have a theory, not totally without foundation, that certain words, which can be used to describe a health disorder, have a powerfully negative effect on the body, not unlike a spell or curse. The word "cancer," for instance, will not go un-noticed by the flesh, and this diagnosis may sign a death sentence within the cells, in the same way that a bone pointed by an aboriginal witch doctor can kill his victim—superstition has merely become more sophisticated, that's all. The words *candida albicans* (when accepted at all by modern medicine) will leave patients with the knowledge that they have one of many "virtually incurable" diseases; this diagnosis does nothing but incite fear. Drug free, dietary alternatives are often so exclusive as to leave the patient weaker, allowing the candida yeast to take over the severely weakened host.

Candida is not a new thing; its symptoms have appeared wherever there has been stress, poor diet, or excess sugar consumption—what is new is that we have given it a name and used that name, often indiscriminately, to sum up a collection of symptoms.

In Victorian times frail "ladies" who were forced by fashion to eat minimally and "sweetly," to wear tight girdles, and avoid sunshine on their "milk white skin" were prone to "the vapours" (not dissimilar in its symptoms to candida or even M.E.).

From an Eastern (oriental) perspective candida, like so many other western disorders, is an example of "damp spleen" or "spleen qi depletion" (or both). This simple assessment contains within it a solution: we need to tonify the spleen or reduce damp creating foods from the diet—a holistic diagnosis that gives the patients the opportunity to assist in their own recovery.

Causes: Like most modern disorders *candida albicans* is usually caused or aggravated by such factors as poor diet (refined rather than whole foods) or inappropriate diets. In England, where candida is rife, diet follows certain fashion trends leading us to often follow the recommended fad diets of warmer, drier climes (such as Southern California or Australia). A diet comprised of tropical fruits, juices, and salad is not a good idea in a country plagued for many months of the year by cold and damp—these foods create an ideal breeding ground for yeast moulds and fungal infections. Excess sugar consumption (the average western person consumes approximately 200 grams of sugar per day, about half of this is sufficient to lower the immune function by up to sixty percent) will also feed internal yeast moulds, exacerbating the problem. Stress and the inappropriate or excessive use of antibiotics will also lower immune function giving rise to a lowered resistance to disease.

Treating Candida with Diet and Herbs

The Chinese consider *candida albicans* to be a condition caused by "excessive damp" of the spleen; they treat it by warming and stimulating the digestive system, whilst eliminating excess fluid. Where there is excess dampness, there is a tendency for fungal or yeast infections to develop, or for water to become "stagnant" giving rise to digestive problems and toxicity in the joints and skin tissues.

In India the most effective treatment for candida follows the above principles using a warming carminative mixture known as *Hingashtak churna*. The American herbalist Michael Tierra has further developed the *Hingashtak* formula, by adding Chinese and western herbs (atractylodes, dandelion root, and slippery elm) to the original Indian spice mix (asafoetida, ginger, caraway, cumin, long pepper, black pepper) making it extremely effective in the treatment of candida, indigestion, and bloating.

Chinese herbalists and Indian vedyas agree that the stomach is where all disease begins, so it is essential to eat sensibly, avoiding too much sugar and cold or raw foods.

THREE USEFUL DIETARY APPROACHES

1) KIDGEREE: Is a traditional Indian food, made from rice and mung beans cooked together with mild spices such as coriander, cumin, and turmeric, with the addition of a little kombu seaweed and ghee. Western alternatives may replace the mung with yellow fish or egg as alternative proteins. But Indian Kidgeree provides a complete protein food and can be eaten as a main meal; cooked vegetables may be added as required.

2) KUDZU: Is a root starch, useful for settling digestion and providing a light carbohydrate source. Kudzu can either be dissolved in cold water and added to the cooking of stir-fried vegetables, or it can be cooked with twig tea and the flesh of an umeboshi plum as a medicinal drink.

3) CONGEE: The Chinese take many of their herbal preparations in the form of soup (or congee). Tonic herbs such as ginseng, codonopsis, and astragalus can be made into a decoction and cooked with rice into a thin gruel.

CHAPTER EIGHT

The Lung: "The Princess of Organs"

JUST AS IN *THE PRINCESS AND THE PEA* story or the story of *Goldilocks*, the lung likes everything to be "just right:" not too wet and not too dry, not too hot and not too cold.

According to Chinese philosophy the lung houses the "corporeal soul" (Po), which dies with the body. The "Wei Qi" (protective or defensive energy), which is ruled by the lung, lives within the skin. The lungs are associated with the ability to receive and let go (as in breathing). Grief (the inability to let go) is connected with lung malfunction, as is the inability to receive gifts and praise.

- The lungs rule Qi (lung Qi descends).
- The lungs move and adjust the water channels (lower oedema, perspiration, urinary issues).
- The lungs govern the externals (skin, hair, etc.).
- The lungs open into the throat (breathing and throat problems).
- The lungs govern the voice (a weak voice indicates either weak lungs or weak kidney Qi).

Lung Dreams: Dreams of flying and seeing strange objects made of gold or iron (metal is the element of the lung), bloody killings, and battle or war (the Samurai, the defenders of justice, are often associated with the lung or protective Qi).

Examples of Lung Imbalance

1. DEFICIENT LUNG QI:

Symptoms: Weak voice, fatigue, weak pulse, shallow breath, white complexion.

Causes: Antibiotics affect lung Qi, suppressive drugs can lead to various disorders including asthma, sarcoidosis and T.B.

Herbs: American Ginseng, Astragalus, Liquorice, etc.

2. LUNG YIN DEFICIENCY:

Symptoms: Dry cough, red tongue (peeled). Heat in the afternoon or evening.

Causes: An irregular diet consumes Yin. The lung is the mother of the kidneys. If the kidneys are weak, they (like a neglected child) can pull on the energy of the mother (the lung).

Herbs: Comfrey, loquat, fritillaria, etc.

Herbs for the Lungs

1) MULLEIN (*verbascum thapsus*, "Aaron's Rod," "Old Man's Flannel," "Velvet Plant," "Candlewick Plant," Great Mullein)

History: Mullein was used by Dioscorides 2,000 years ago to treat lung conditions.

Folklore & Legend: Mullein is used in India to protect from evil. Native American peoples use the flower stalk as an incense to protect their homes. In the European classics Mullein was used by Ulysses to protect himself from the seductions of Circe.

"Mullein" is the Latin term for leprosy or "mallandrium." It was a very popular herb in medieval Europe.

Actions: Expectorant, analgesic.

Ruler: Saturn.

Uses: The demulcent, emollient, and astringent properties of mullein make it useful for the treatment of coughs, bronchitis, asthma, hay fever, dyspnoea, sinusitis, swollen glands, lung infections, mumps, and internal bleeding of both lungs and

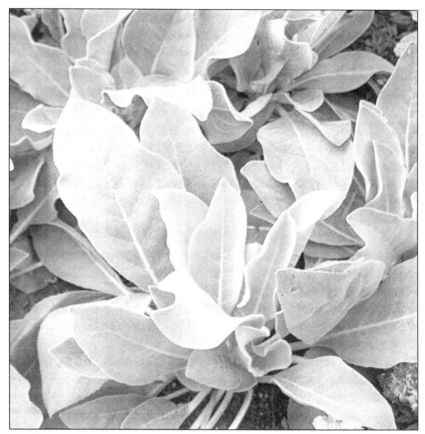

PLATE 4. Mullein.

intestines. Mullein will dispel heat and congestion from the lungs and nasal passages (the leaves used as steam inhalation). The plant also has slight sedative and narcotic properties.

Mullein flowers have strong nervine, anti-inflammatory, and analgesic properties. Used in a Macerated oil, mullein can be useful in treating piles, bruising, and earache.

Mullein juice or fresh flowers are recommended in the treatment of warts. Greek fisherman used the seeds of some members of the verbascum family to intoxicate fish, and another member of the same family was used in Madeira to expel tapeworms.

51

The epithet "Thapsus" is believed to have been derived from either the Greek settlement of Thapsos in Sicily or the Tunisian city of Thapsus. Mullein is found growing in both locations.

N.B. If Mullein leaves and flowers are used as tea for coughs, etc., it must be well strained to remove irritating leaf hairs.

2) COMFREY ROOT (*Symphytum officinale*, "knitbone")

Comfrey root has demulcent, expectorant properties and is extremely high in mucilage making it a useful herb in the treatment of dry coughs (such as whooping cough) and conditions involving internal bleeding (either from the lungs or stomach).

It is generally considered that the true comfrey officinale has white or cream flowers, whereas the common purple flowering comfrey is slightly inferior in terms of medicinal use. Comfrey Root contains the substance allanton, a cell proliferant known to speed up the natural replacement of body cells, making this herb useful in treating many conditions from burns to broken bones.

The medicinal use of comfrey root was restricted in Europe due to some pretty flawed research. Symphytine, an active ingredient in comfrey root, has been shown to cause cancer in rats that were injected with the pure alkaloid in high doses[13] (I know of no one who would consider injecting him or herself with an active ingredient of comfrey). Two cases of liver toxicity due to comfrey use have been reported in the US. I am only able to find information on one of these: a woman drank up to ten cups of comfrey tea a day while taking handfuls of comfrey pills over a period of more than a year (a hardly surprising result under the circumstances).

Comfrey grows extremely fast, and its leaves can be harvested three or four times a year and rotted down as a high nutrient plant feed. The young leaves of comfrey are high in Vitamin B12; they can be fried in batter as tempura or lightly steamed as greens (used in moderation).

3) ELECAMPANE (*Inula helenium, elfswort, pushkaramula, hsuan fu hua*)

Elecampane is one of the best rejuvenatives for the lungs, absorbing water, and reducing swelling. It has a calming effect on the digestive system, the mind, and female reproductive system.

Folklore: Both Pliny and Dioscorides claimed that the external use of the root hairs would cure snakebite.

Active Ingredients: Elecampane contains high amounts of Inula, thought to be useful as a sweetener for diabetics.

Actions: Expectorant, carminative, analgesic, and rejuvenative.

Indications: Colds, asthma, and nervous disability.

N.B. Avoid with hot conditions.

4) OSHA (*ligusticum porterii*, "mountain ginseng," "bear medicine," "Colorado cough root")

Osha is an herb in the umbellifera family used by Native American peoples to purify the environment, and it is highly regarded as a medicine. Its name "bear medicine" refers to the fact that sick bears, or bears recovering from the weakening effects of long periods of hibernation, eat large quantities of this root (Echinacea angustifolia is similarly called "Elk root" due to elks being attracted to it during times of sickness).

Actions: Anti-viral, carminative, diaphoretic, diuretic, immune stimulant, mildly anaesthetic (in cases of toothache, etc.).

Uses: Sore throats, coughs, respiratory infections, fevers, diarrhoea.[14] I personally find Osha to be one of the best herbs to use in cases of stubborn coughs, as it appears to dissolve stubborn mucous and combines well with mullein, grindelia, and other herbs for the lung.

Many plants in the ligusticum genus are used in herbal medicine. Chuan Xiong (*ligusticum wallichii, Szechuan lovage*) has been used in China for more than 800 years for amenorrhoea and dysmenorrhoea, headaches and thrombosis.[15] Chuan Xiong is a key herb in the Chinese formula Si Wu Tang (Four materials decoction).

Osha is not easy to cultivate, as its growth is dependent on a particular fungus in the soil. Care should be taken when harvesting to assure correct identification (many umbelliferic plants are toxic) and to not over-harvest (in 1993 Osha was listed as "rare" but has not yet been listed as "endangered").

General Herbs for Treating Lung Conditions

AMERICAN GINSENG: Demulcent tonic.

APRICOT SEED: Cough, asthma, bronchitis.

ASPARAGUS: Lung dryness.

ASTRAGALUS: Strengthens immune system.

BALM OF GILEAD: Anti-inflammatory.

CAYENNE: Circulatory stimulant.

COMFREY Rt.: Dry cough, inflammation.

ECHINACEA: Immune stimulant.

ELECAMPANE: Soothes coughs, prevents infection.

EUCALYPTUS: Powerful antiseptic.

FRITILLARY: Bronchitis, asthma, etc.

GRINDELLIA: Stimulates repair of lung tissues, liquefies mucous, aids expectoration.

HONEYSUCKLE: Reduces infection and inflammation.

HYSSOP: Treats sore throats and lung congestion.

LIQUORICE: Soothes mucous membranes.

LOBELIA: Contains lobeline a powerful respiratory stimulant, which works on the same receptor sites as nicotine, helps with nicotine withdrawal symptoms. (Lobelia's use is restricted in both Europe and Australia.)

LOQUAT: Expels phlegm, clears inflammation.

MARSHMALLOW: Soothes inflamed throat tissues.

MULLEIN: Relieves bronchial irritation.

OPHIOPOGON: For dry cough and T.B.

OSHA: Bronchial dilator stimulates removal of mucous from the lungs.

PIPPLI: Dries mucous.

PLATYCODON: Loosens phlegm.

PROPOLIS: Slows down tissue degradation.

REISHI: Immune stimulant inhibits histamine release.

STILLINGIA: Increases lymph drainage treats bronchial inflammation.

THYME: For chronic respiratory infections.

WILD CHERRY: Acts as a mild sedative to mucous membranes.

WILD INDIGO: Tones defence system.

YERBA SANTA: Shrinks inflamed tissue.

Key Formula for Lung: Yu Ping Feng Wan (Jade Screen)

Yu ping feng wan is the most recommended Chinese herbal formula for building resistance against infection. This formula (commonly known as "Jade Screen" or "Jade Windscreen Powder") is useful in protecting a weakened immune system from viral or bacterial attack (or what the Chinese refer to as "external evils"). Chinese health authorities recommended Jade Screen during the SARS outbreak, and research has found it to be useful in protecting against the H5NI flu virus. The main ingredients in Jade Screen are Astragalus, Siler, and Atractylodes.

In Chinese Medicine the lung tends to relate to the Western concept of an "Immune System." Lung Qi is seen as a protective umbrella, which guards the body from "external evils."

John E. Smith

Natural Immunity

When antibiotics first appeared on the medical scene, it was thought that immune system disorders would be a thing of the past. These disorders, which now include M.E., A.I.D.S., and a whole battalion of new health problems, are greatly on the increase and often fatal. Reduced immune function now appears to be caused by many new factors including: indiscriminate use of antibiotics, cortisol steroids, vaccines, contraceptive pills, chemotherapy, X-Rays, and environmental pollutants (the average city dweller now takes in 2 kilos of such pollutants each year).

DIET: Is an important factor in maintaining balanced immune function. The diet needs to be rich in anti-oxidants (such as Vitamin C, A, E, Zinc and Selenium, etc.) with the avoidance of excessive use of refined sugars, dairy products, yeast, vinegar, red meat, saturated fats, caffeine, nicotine, and alcohol.

STRESS: Creates adrenal weakness and resulting fatigue. Stress is largely caused by excess stimulation and can be treated by rest, relaxation, meditation, gentle exercise (including yoga, Tai Chi, etc.), sedatives, adaptogenic herbs, or nervine tonic herbs (such as passiflora, chamomile, valerian, etc.). There are a great many eastern adaptogens, which are particularly effective in reducing the effects of stress. These include: Gotu Kola (*hydrocotyl asiatica*), Zyziphus (Chinese red date seeds), Schizandra (*S.Chinensis*), and Eleuthero (*E. sentinococcus*). Eleuthero (Siberian Ginseng) not only reduces stress but also enhances the immune system.

OTHER IMMUNE SYSTEM HERBS INCLUDE:

Echinacea: An herb with strong antibiotic properties, which stimulates natural killer cells and initiates the production of interferon (a cell protein useful in treating tumours, etc.).

Garlic: Contains certain compounds that bind to heavy metals, rendering them harmless.

Liquorice: Anti-viral, immune stimulating strengthens adrenal glands.

Shitake: An edible mushroom used in Japanese hospitals to treat stomach cancer.

Reishi: One of the most effective medicinal mushrooms in the treatment of immune disorders.

Yerba Santa Leaf: Known by early Spanish settlers in America as "Holy Weed" or "Consumptives Weed." Yerba Santa is known to stimulate salivary glands and shrink inflamed tissue. Yerba Santa is a leading agent for all respiratory conditions.

I also feel a need to mention a few lesser-known herbs, which stand a great chance of becoming very popular as immune systems become more compromised and some of the more popular herbs (such as Golden Seal) become unavailable due to over-harvesting.

1) IGDE: (*Oleaster, eleagnus*, "silverberry tree," "Russian olive")

High in antioxidants and lycopene.

Effective against cancer (undocumented).

Grows throughout Middle East, Asia and Orient.

Attractive to bees, birds and butterflies.

I recently came across perfume oil made from the seeds and flowers of this herb; it is an exquisite perfume with an uplifting fragrance.

I would be grateful for more information on this herb, so if anyone can help, please e-mail me (jesmithbodytonix@aol.com).

2) MOUNTAIN TEA: (*Sideritis* "Iron wort," "Olympus tea," "Shepherd's tea")

History: In the first century A.D. Dioscorides discovered this herb when he travelled throughout the Mediterranean with Roman legions and studied the benefits of the plants he encountered.

Active Ingredients: Mountain Tea is very rich in flavinoids.

Actions: Anti-inflammatory, anti-oxidant.

Uses: Common cold, flu, allergies, respiratory problems and digestion. General Immune system support.

3) DITTANY: Known as Dittany of Crete, Spanish hops, and erada (meaning love).

There are three different types of dittany—this one is from the oregano family.

It is hermaphrodite (both organs are pollinated by bees).

History: Used by Hippocrates for treating stomach problems, poor digestion, rheumatism and menstrual issues.

Uses: To heal wounds, soothe pain, ease childbirth. The juice was traditionally used to treat snakebite. Combined with cinnamon and honey for coughs.

Folklore: In "the language of flowers" dittany relates to passion and is used ritually as an ingredient in incense. In medieval witchcraft dittany was an important ingredient in "Flying Ointment" (no current research to back its effectiveness). Legend claims it protects from piercing by arrows, and it was used in the Trojan wars as a poultice for wounds and the removal of embedded arrows.[16]

4) JUNIPER: Is another great herb, which deserves a mention.

Juniper is described by several traditions as "The Great Protector" and considered by many herbal authorities to be a key herb in protecting the immune system from pandemics such as Avian Flu.

Juniper is considered a protecting herb in cultures as far apart as Tibet and The Navajo Nation. Its key word as an alchemical spagyric essence and in "the language of flowers" is "protection." Its Latin name *Juniperus Communis* points to its potential use in Community medicine, e.g., epidemics and pandemics.

Tobacco: *Its Use and Abuse*

Tobacco abuse is currently the greatest underlying causes of death in the United Kingdom. Mortality statistics in 1991 showed it to be responsible for an estimated 110,000 deaths that year alone. The immunologist, Richard Petts, has stated that according to current trends, smoking will claim 500 million lives (world wide) in the next twenty-five years. Research in Pennsylvania has shown that heavy smoking can cut an average of eighteen years from a normal lifespan.

Tobacco is a noxious weed that (according to historians) was imported from the Americas by Sir Walter Raleigh in 1586. Raleigh's journal entries (referring to how smoking the weed encouraged laughter and dancing) might actually indicate that he brought back the wrong herb (or in street terminology "was sold a bum deal"). If Raleigh had brought back the herb referred to in his journal, the British may have been more relaxed, but it is also likely that the country may have ground to a total stand-still a few centuries ago.

French historians claim tobacco was first introduced into Europe in 1559 by Jean Nicot, (whose name was given to the active ingredient "nicotine," a poison as effective as *curare*).

MEDICINAL USES: Tobacco is useful as an emetic. It works harshly so should be used in emergencies by those with a strong constitution. Some years ago in Australia I was able to witness the latter use: A cattle dog had taken a poisoned bait; an Aboriginal man I knew forced the dog to swallow a large wodge of tobacco. He then swung the dog (by its tail) around his head until it vomited up the poison—a good example of "Bush Medicine."

Tobacco is also a good medicine against rheumatic pains and can be used in ointments to treat inflamed haemorrhoids. A mild infusion will kill head-lice and distilled oil can be used for toothache (with a great deal of care—pure nicotine is lethal). Chewed and mixed with saliva, tobacco has been applied to snakebites with some success.

John E. Smith

"As to the practice of chewing or taking as snuff,
little can be said for them from practice, and nothing
from reason: nor much for smoking. If these customs
had any good tendency, it would be taken off by the
constant practice."

—Hill's Family Herbal.

ANTIDOTES: Chewing cloves after a cigarette will remove the taste and reduce the desire to smoke. Gotu kola, calamus and celery seeds all act as antidotes to nicotine and may help to reduce dependency. Magnolia tea is useful in handling tobacco addiction, as is lobelia. Various herbs can be taken as tea to help cleanse and settle the system whilst undergoing withdrawal. These include: slippery elm, vervain, peppermint, burdock root, black cohosh, and echinacea.

Breaking the Tobacco Habit

Apart from the use of the herbs previously mentioned, breaking habits obviously require conscious effort and commitment.

Smoke Consciously: Before lighting your next cigarette ask yourself, WHY? Is it a reflex action? Because you are with other smokers, you are nervous, or because you always smoke with a cup of tea or after a meal. Ask your lungs, "Do you really want this cigarette?" If you decide to go ahead anyway, then smoke alone, in the open air, without tea or any other associated stimulation; be totally aware of the action of smoking. Then ask your lungs, "Well how do you feel now?" Practice conscious smoking for a while, note the results, and see how much more easily you are able to cut down.

LIGHT HEARTED WARNING!

"When things really get too bad on the planet Earth
and it starts to fall apart from wars and pollution and

*earthquakes and so forth, then Higher Beings are
going to come in flying saucers and rescue the more
evolved souls among us; but they can't take smokers
aboard their spaceships because people with nicotine
in their systems explode when they enter the seventh
dimension."*
 —*Even Cowgirls Get the Blues,* Tom Robbins.

10 STEPS TO GIVING UP SMOKING:
1. You must want to give up smoking forever and be able to verbalize this, otherwise there is no point.
2. Reduce gradually, dividing the waking day into segments of three hours; allow yourself so many cigarettes in each segment of time (no storing, or borrowing from other time segments). Reduce this allowance over a designated period of time.
3. Specify a stopping date, and work towards this by gradually reducing the number of cigarettes smoked.
4. Smoke only in designated areas.
5. Smoke consciously. Really think about every cigarette and ask yourself, "Do I need (rather than 'do I want') this cigarette." After smoking, ask yourself how much you really enjoyed the cigarette on a scale of one to ten.
6. Use smoking substitutes. Liquorice root is a good one; it can be bought in pieces roughly the same size as a cigarette. This provides a way of occupying the hands while having a soothing action on previously damaged mucous membranes.
7. Start using the sense of smell more—smell flowers, food, air, etc. See how unpleasant clothing, hair, and fingers smell after smoking.
8. Build up a network of supportive friends who you can talk to when cravings strike.
9. Use herbs and natural therapies, which help to detoxify the system and reduce cravings.
10. CONGRATULATIONS!

John E. Smith

P.S. Major Tobacco Companies include an average of 599 additives in cigarettes including: Aconitic acid, Ammonia, Civet absolute, Acetate, Phosphoric acid, flour, and sugar.

CHAPTER NINE

The Kidneys & Adrenals: "The Storehouse of Energy"

"The mansion of fire and water, the channel of life and death."

IN TRADITIONAL CHINESE MEDICINE (TCM) the adrenals are included in with the kidneys rather than treated as separate organs. The adrenals are referred to as the "Yang" aspect and the kidneys themselves as the "Yin" aspect.

According to TCM:

- The kidneys are the basis of pre-natal life (kidney deficiency will cause premature ageing).
- The kidneys store the "vital essence" (their affliction affects the "in breath").
- The kidneys control the bones (including the teeth) and communicate with the brain.
- The kidney channels open to the ear.
- Flourishing of the kidneys shows in the hair.
- The kidneys control urination, defecation, and fluid balance.
- The kidney is the root of ancestral or congenital Qi.

Symptoms of Imbalance: Lower back pain, joint pains, weakness of lower extremities (especially the knees), urinary problems, fatigue, loose teeth, bone weakness, hearing problems, and impotence.

KIDNEY YANG DEFICIENCY:

Symptoms: (at least three of the following)—Coldness, pale complexion, clear urine, night sweats, oedema, pale thick tongue, weak deep pulse.

Mode of Treatment: Warm and Tonify Kidney Yang.

Herbs: Cinnamon bark, epemidium, walnut kernels, fenugreek, etc.

KIDNEY YIN DEFICIENCY:

Symptoms: (at least three of the following)—Lack of essence, infertility, no menstrual cycle, poor memory, premature ageing, hair loss, loose teeth, weak knees, slowness, lack of fire.

Mode of Treatment: Nourish Kidney Yin.

Herbs: Rehmannia, fo-ti, shatavari, juniper, etc.

Good Foods for the Kidneys

Black Morello Cherry: Juice will tonify kidney Qi and help with urinary problems, as will cranberry juice.

Pork: (well cooked) is a good kidney tonic, cooked with cornus, schizandra, Chinese yam, and cinnamon.

Salt: Salty foods, such as fetta cheese, seaweeds, olives, etc., will tonify kidneys and adrenals (used in moderation)—Salt cravings will be a symptom of adrenal exhaustion.

Seeds: All seeds (including grains, pulses, etc.) will generally tonify the "seed energy" of the kidneys.

FOODS BEST AVOIDED: Excessive amounts of salt (see above) and excessive amounts of stimulants such as coffee, cola, guarana, etc. (Guarana may "kick start" the adrenals, but will exhaust them in the long term.)

Herbs for the Kidneys & Bladder

1) EUCOMMIA: (Du Zhong, euccommia ulmoides)

Eucommia bark always reminds me of snakeskin with its elastically separated sections, indicating its common use in strengthening the spine and improving joint flexibility.

History: First mentioned in *The Divine Husbandman's Classic* of the Materia Medica (Chinese Han Dynasty).

Specific Use: Deficient Kidney Yang.

Symptoms: High blood pressure, pale face, feelings of coldness, lower back pain, knee weakness, oedema, frequent urination.

Other Uses: Eucommia can be used to calm the foetus in cases of cold deficiency and bleeding during pregnancy. The bark can be cooked with salt water to increase its potency—a small amount of salt will take the energy of the herb to the kidneys.

Toxicity: No cases of toxicity or overdose recorded.

2) EPEMIDIUM: ("Horny Goat Weed")

Horny Goat Weed supposedly gained its title from the observations of an ancient Chinese goatherd who noticed the increased amorous activity of his goats when grazing on the weed. Apparently it can be as beneficial to women as well as men (and goats).

Epimedium (otherwise known in the West as Barrenwort or in China as Yin Yang Huo) is part of the *Berberidaceae* family of hardy perennials. It is a long valued kidney and adrenal tonic in traditional Chinese herbalism. It was first recorded in the *Shen Non Ben Cao Jing* in about 200 B.C.—100 A.D. and has long been observed to have aphrodisiac qualities with the key constituent being observed to be icariin.

Modern studies in China with animals seem to show that Epimedium stimulates endocrine secretions of a type of androgen (substances like androsterone and testosterone that stimulate male characteristics) by relaxing smooth muscle (probably with increased levels of nitric oxide) and increasing erectile function.

3) CINNAMON BARK: (*Cinnamomum zeylanicum, Rou Gui***).** A stimulant, astringent, carminative, used to warm the body and aid circulation, also useful in lower back pain or weakness and as a digestive aid. The bark is used in Chinese medicine to treat the trunk of the body, whereas the twig (gui zhi) is used to "release the exterior" by opening the pores.

Active constituents: Essential oil, mucilage, sucrose, and resin. Cinnamon bark also contains the chemical cinnamaldehyde, known to destroy E Coli, Salmonella, and Staphylococcus aurea. Cinnameldehyde also has a mildly tranquillising effect, which helps reduce anxiety.

Indications: Indigestion, gas, poor circulation, rheumatism, colds, flu, lower back and heart pain, impotence.

Precautions: Not to be taken in higher doses during pregnancy.

Cinnamon is a potent stimulant, which works primarily on the kidneys and adrenals; it has a warming effect, increasing vitality, clearing congestion, and aiding circulation. Cinnamon helps to enhance the immune function and improve the ability to withstand stress.

Folklore and Traditional Use: Pliny (first century A.D.) records how the price of cinnamon was raised by the rumour that it was protected by "a terrible kind of bat."

The best Vietnamese cinnamon bark is a very expensive herb to this day.

4) SOLIDAGO: (Solidago virgurea, Golden Rod, "Blue Mountain Tea")

"Sovereign wound herb of particular efficacy in all lotions for sores and ulcers in the mouth, throat or privities of either sex."

—Culpepper

Golden Rod is an attractive garden plant, thought to bring good luck when grown near the home.

Ruler: Venus.

Actions: Diuretic, anti-inflammatory, anti-spasmodic, antiseptic.

Uses: Solidago strengthens kidney function and counters irritation caused by either infection or kidney stones. It will also help in dissolving stones and gravel in the urinary tract and removing the toxins that are often responsible for some skin conditions. Solidago is also thought to reduce the amount of calcium build-up in the kidneys and thereby lessen the formation of stones.

The Latin word Solidago (using an aspect of "the doctrine of signatures") can be said to strengthen or "solidify" us in the past (*ago*). The organs behind us are, of course, the kidneys. In spagyric medicine Solidago is actually used to remedy problems caused in the distant past.

Key Formula: *Rehmania Six*

Historical Antecedents: *Liu Wei Di Huang Wan*—6 Flavour Rehmannia Pill, *Ming Mu Di Huang Wan*—Bright Eyes Shining Pill—*Er Ming Zuo Ci Wan*—Ear Ringing Left Loving Pill.

Rehmannia Six is a slightly modified version of at least three classical yin-nourishing formulas from Chinese medicine (see above). This formula is ideal for people who constantly over extend themselves and become exhausted due to irregular or skipped meals and insufficient rest.

Simple Assessment Guide: (any three of the following)—A person who is thin, dry, wasted, with insomnia, low back pain or weakness, night sweats, high blood pressure, diabetes, eye disorders, tinnitus.

Traditional Use: Classical approach to nourishing kidney, liver and spleen yin, including such symptoms as empty heat with night sweats and dizziness, heat in palm of hands and soles of feet, ringing in ears, glaucoma, impotence, and diabetes.

Safety: This formula can be used long term, but caution should be taken in cases of extreme dampness and poor digestion.

CHAPTER TEN

The Liver: "The General of the Army"

- The liver rules the flow of energy in the body; it controls the nerves and the sub-costal region.
- The liver stores the blood and its malfunction can therefore be responsible for menstrual disorders.
- Because the liver controls the ligaments, loss of grasp in the hands and even epilepsy can be seen as liver deficiency.
- The liver opens into the eyes, impaired vision is often associated with poor liver function.
- The liver governs the power of regeneration, birth, inspiration, and creativity.

General Symptoms of Liver Imbalance

IN EXCESS:

Stuffiness of chest, sub costal pain, anger, restlessness, vertigo, red-face, bowstring pulse, spasms.

IN DEFICIENCY:

Symptoms: Pallor, insomnia, dreams, dry eyes, poor sight, numbness of limbs, convulsions, pale tongue.

DEFICIENT LIVER YIN:

Symptoms: Headache, small rapid bowstring pulse.

Healing Principle: Nourish liver blood.

Herbs: Lycium, peony alba, rehmannia, dong quai.

STAGNATION OF LIVER QI:

Symptoms: Chest stagnation, bloating and pain in lower abdomen, irregular menstrual cycle, lumps in abdomen, uneven bowstring pulse.

Healing Principle: Move stagnation.

Herbs: Bupleurum, peony, liquorice.

LIVER YANG UPRISING:

Symptoms: Restlessness, anger, pain in head and eyes, deafness, red-face, red eyes, heavy nasal breathing, scanty yellow urine, dry faeces, yellow tongue fur, rapid pulse, shout.

Healing Principle: Dispel Fire.

Herbs: Raw Rehmannia, peony, pearl, oyster shell.

FOODS BEST AVOIDED:

The liver is adversely affected by:

    a.   Toxins from alcohol.
    b.   Stimulants (such as coffee).
    c.   The use of chemical drugs or toxic plants (whether prescribed or non-prescribed).
    d.   Nut oils and animal fats.

Key Herb: White Peony—(*bai shao yao,* peony alba, p.lactiflora)

Peony root is commonly used in many liver formulas in Chinese medicine, particularly those relating to hormonal and menstrual imbalances in women.

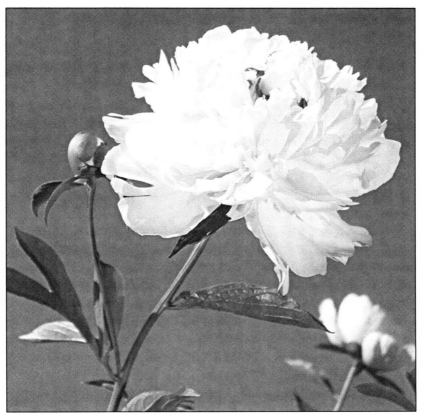

PLATE 5.   White Peony.

Peony is a key herb in formulae such as "four treasures" (*si wu tang*), "8 precious herbs" (*ba zhen wan*), and "Free and Easy Wanderer" (*xiao yao wan*). It is used to move qi (energy), nourish the blood, and harmonise the functions of liver and spleen.

Actions: Antispasmodic, analgesic, sedative, astringent, and emmenagogue.

Uses: Irregular menses, abdominal spasm, headaches, night sweats, disharmony of liver and spleen, to pacify liver.

Red Peony: Improves blood circulation.

71

John E. Smith

Key Formula for the Liver: Xiao Yao Wan— ("Free & Easy Wanderer")

Traditional Use: To nourish liver yin and blood, invigorate congested liver qi, harmonise liver and stomach-spleen.

Major Organ System: The Liver is the organ that deals with almost everything that enters the body, whether physical (foods, toxins, etc.), mental (thoughts, mental pressure, etc.), or emotional (worries, feelings, stress, etc.). When unable to deal with these pressures immediately, the liver (due to its nature as a storage organ) will put them aside for later processing; this can often result in "stuckness" or "stagnant qi."

Stagnant Qi is expressed by such symptoms as tightness of neck, shoulders and breasts, headaches, fatigue, poor digestion, and moods such as frustration or depression. Xiao yao wan— cleanses the liver by moving "stuck qi" allowing its function to return to normal. This formula is a useful adjunct to treating most disorders including menstrual and digestive imbalances (such as infertility, PMS, abdominal bloating, and poor appetite). Xiao yao wan is a basic formula for stagnation of liver qi due to deficiency of liver blood.

Ingredients: Chinese Angelica, Bupleurum, Atractylodes, White Peony, Ginger, Poria Cocos, Liquorice, and Mint.

CHAPTER ELEVEN

Ayurveda: "The Science of Life."

"Herbs that sprang up in time of old, three ages earlier than the Gods,

Of these, whose hue is brown, will I declare the hundred powers and seven.

Ye, Mothers, have a hundred homes, yea, and a thousand are your growths.

Do ye who have a thousand powers free this my patient from disease.

Be glad and joyful in the Plants, both blossoming and bearing fruit,

Plants that will lead us to success like mares who conquer in the race."

—Taken from Rig Veda, tenth Mandalla, 1700–1100 B.C.

History & Mythology

No introduction to Ayurveda can be anywhere near complete without examining its roots and some of the Vedic myths and legends that inspire its teachings.

Veda can loosely be translated as "knowledge" or "wisdom" and refers to the historical texts of Hinduism. There are four main "Vedas" or Vedic texts with numerous subtexts and commentaries.

Rig Veda is considered the earliest (1700–1100 B.C.); it is comprised of 1028 hymns in ten cycles (mandalas). These hymns are memorized and passed down by the Hotri Priests.

Sama Veda, the tunes or songs, is passed down by the Udgatri Priests.

Yajur Veda, the sacrifices, is the domain of the Arvaryu Priests.

Atharva (artha translates roughly as "goal") or the spells, belong to the Atharvans. It is from Atharva Veda that the philosophy of Ayurveda is drawn.

The Brahmin Priests became the custodians of the mantras and many of the earlier texts, which became translated into written form, these became described as the Brahmanas and included such texts as *The Laws of Manu* (300 B.C.) and various Vedic Commentaries. Spoken commentaries and rites (between 800–200 B.C.) included the Aranyakas (forest passages) and The Upanishads (literally "To sit down near") or secret teachings. The Aranyakas were the manifestation of "internal religion" and the Upanishads were the discussions between seers and their disciples.

Hindu Myths (Itihasas) provide us with interesting stories regarding creation and mankind's search for immortality—A key element of Ayurvedic Medicine.

In the beginning of this world cycle, the formless one was floating on a timeless milk ocean. The night of Brahma was coming to a close, and from within the formlessness there stirred the seed of creation. The seed sprouted from the navel of the Absolute and became a thousand petal lotus. In the lotus Brahma meditated on his next cosmic drama. The play needed a plot, which would encompass a cycle of 8,640 million years. However much Brahma tried, the plot would not come; there

was only one word, one unifying vibration, and the play of creation demanded multiplicity.

Brahma meditated for a thousand years, until each of his thoughts had the power of spontaneous manifestation; each name automatically became form. The plot of Brahma's play was immortality.

In order for the play to continue for the prescribed duration Brahma needed to hide the nectar of immortality from his creations (the gods, demons and humans, who were actors in his play). Brahma took the ambrosia and hid it at the bottom of the ocean, but the gods and demons (normally at war) became united by a common desire to churn up the ocean. The ocean was churned with the Mandara Mountain, around which Ananta, the world serpent, was coiled as a rope. Vishnu, in his second incarnation as a tortoise, steadied the mountain at its base, for it is the nature of Vishnu to maintain support and balance from the underlying field of existence.

When the ambrosia was found, Garuda, the giant man-eagle or phoenix, took it to Indra, the king of the gods. The archer, Krishanu, tried to shoot Garuda but only succeeded in dislodging a single feather, which fell to the earth as lightning.

Garuda spilled a few drops of the ambrosia on the grass and the serpents greedily licked them up. Garuda was granted immortality when he returned the moon to the gods.[17]

So Brahma again took the nectar and hid it in the highest Himalayas . . .

Hanuman, the monkey god, was sent by Rama and his brother Lakshman (wounded in battle) to seek an immortal herb. So Hanuman meditated on Mount Mahendra until he became the size of the mountain. He was unsure which herb to bring back so returned with the entire mountain. This delayed his return, and the moon had started to rise. Hanuman knew that the herb would be ineffective if exposed to moonlight, so he ate the moon.

On his return, he was offered a boon by Rama and chose to live as long as men spoke of Rama's deeds. He thus attained immortality. Rama reigned as King of Ayodhya for 10,000 years and his story, The Ramayana, became one of the major Hindu epics.

The Yogis and ascetics, in their search for solitude, climbed the loftiest Himalayan peaks and imbibed the nectar by breathing the air and eating medicinal plants.

"We have drunk Soma, we have become immortal, we have entered into the light, we have known the gods." Vedic Hymn.

Brahma, in fear that the entire universe would return to the oneness of his own immortal nature, took the ambrosia and plunged it deep within mankind. He knew that there it would be safe for all time, for it is the nature of man to look outside of himself, never seeing the kingdom within.

Authors Note: *The above story is my own, and has been drawn from various sources. It is not my aim to present an accurate account, as I was definitely not there at the time. It is my hope that my version of the above stories will not offend serious Vedic scholars. I have a great deal of respect for this ancient tradition of knowledge.*

So goes the story of creation and the search for immortality; it has its parallels in all traditions. The tree of life from the garden of Eden, the Holy Grail, the magic cauldrons of Gaelic and Celtic mythology, the nectar of Greek and Roman legends.

Ayurveda is probably the oldest health system of the world; it came into being in India's "Golden Age" inspired and influenced by the Vedic scriptures, which are considered by devout Hindus to be the "Blueprints of Creation."

Ayurveda (literally translated as "The Wisdom of Life") is one of the four "Upa" (higher) Vedas and covers various disciplines used to "purify" the body (including diet, herbal medicine, and lifestyle recommendations).

Mythology tells us that Ayurveda was first "cognised" by the sage Bharadwaja who passed the knowledge on to Susrut and Charak, who wrote the major texts (samhitas). Susrut is now thought to have been the son of Vishwamitra, the spiritual adviser of King Rama.

Although much of the wisdom of Ayurveda was lost when Alexander invaded India, it was revived by King Ashoka and taken abroad by Buddhist monks and had a later influence on both Chinese and Tibetan Medicine.

Ayurveda uses diet, daily practices, herbs, and mantras to promote harmony and prevent sickness.

"Avert the danger which has not yet come."
—Yogi Patanjali.

Although the primary medicines take the form of foods, elixirs (*rasayanas*) may be herbal or mineral in composition, some containing alchemically processed metals and gemstones. It is considered that medicines can be taken in many forms. If the awareness is pure, even the name of the medicine can be used as a mantra to infuse its value in consciousness, but during sickness the purest form of awareness is difficult to achieve, so we use medicine.

"He who has not fallen sick is Ayurveda."
—Vedya Trigunaji

The major focus of Ayurveda is on digestion, so a great deal of emphasis is placed on food. A patient will be advised to include the six major tastes (rasas) in a diet to maintain the gastric fire (agni).

THE SIX TASTES (RASAS):

Sour: digestant

Salt: cleansing

Pungent: appetising

Bitter: appetising and purifying

Astringent: healing and drying **Sweet:** nourishing

The degree to which each of these tastes will be used will depend on the imbalance of the humours.

The Three Humours or "Tridosha"

The five elements (fire, earth, air, water, and ether) come together in different combinations to form the three humours or "doshas." These doshas are known as Vata (air and ether), Pitta (fire and water), and Kapha (earth and water). Vata, Pitta, and Kapha together govern all the biological and psychological functions of the body; they are the foundation of human existence; they support the body when normal, and destroy it when abnormal.

THE QUALITIES OF THE DOSHAS

Vata is cold, light, dry, mobile, subtle, clear, and astringent.

Pitta is hot, penetrating, oily, sharp, spreading, and sour.

Kapha is slow, heavy, cool, soft, sticky, and liquid.

THE SITES OF THE DOSHAS

Vata is said to reside in the colon, the thighs, the ears and the bones.

Pitta dominates the eyes, the blood, stomach, small intestines, and the grey matter of the brain.

Kapha dominates lymph, muscles, joints, sinuses, lungs, kidneys, connective tissue, etc. (All visible cells, tissues and organs are made up of kapha.)

THE FUNCTIONS OF THE DOSHAS

Vata is responsible for all movement, all sensory functions, and the working of the intellect.

Pitta is the metabolic force of the body. It is responsible for digestion, body temperature, vision, hunger, thirst, taste, complexion, and power of discrimination.

Kapha gives shape, lubricates, provides energy, and protects the heart and lungs. It is the file on which all our experiences of life are stored in the white matter of the brain.

Times and Seasons of Increase of the Doshas

Vata dominates before sunrise and sunset, during summer and autumn, and in old age.

Pitta dominates at noon and midnight, during spring and summer, and in adulthood/middle age.

Kapha dominates after sunrise and sunset, during winter and spring, and in youth/childhood.

RESPONSES

People with a particular dominant dosha will respond to situations according to that dosha. The **Vata Response** will be emotional. The **Pitta Response** will be rational. The **Kapha** person will respond with great consideration.

SYMPTOMS OF DOSHA IMBALANCE

Vata: Emaciation, dryness, fatigue, spasm, constipation, numbness, stiffness, osteoporosis, moving pain, fear/anxiety.

Pitta: Yellowish discolouration, heat, thirst, vomiting, nausea, hives, ulceration, diarrhoea, burning pain, hatred/anger/envy/judgement.

Kapha: Obesity, depression, lethargy, diabetes, oedema, tumours, cough, dull pain.

John E. Smith

Ayurvedic Recipes

*"From torment by threefold misery arises the inquiry
into the means of terminating it."*
—Samkhya Karika 1,1.

Kapha: Honey water in the morning.

Pitta: Pomegranate seeds and juice, with amla and aloe juice.

Vata: 1. Sesame oil, lightly roasted kalonji seeds, with cider vinegar. 2. Chopped garlic preserved for 30 days in sesame oil and rock salt.

HARMONISING RECIPES: *(to balance three doshas)*
1. Red rice cooked with coconut milk and black sesame seeds (dry roasted and ground).
2. Cooked mung beans with pomegranate seeds, live yoghurt, and rock salt.
3. Oily fish with mustard oil and rock salt.
4. Small greenish white aubergines (wild if possible) with black sesame seeds, tamarind, rock salt, and sesame oil. (This can also be used to stuff Karela, bitter gourd).
5. Fenugreek sprouts cooked with spinach and sesame oil.
6. Organic chicken with mustard oil, pomegranate seeds, yoghurt, and rock salt.
7. Mung beans and curry leaves, sesame seeds, rock salt, fresh ginger, and tamarind.
8. Garlic cooked with buttermilk, date sugar, cumin, coriander, asafoetida, turmeric, and rock salt.

Fasting Tea (to harmonise doshas): Ingredients: 4 parts violet leaves (or gotu kola or chickweed), 1 part black peppercorns, 1 part anise seeds, 1 part rose petals.

Method: 1 oz of herb mix to 1 pint of water, steep 15 minutes in boiling water and strain, mix with equal amount of warm milk and a little honey.

Organ Rejuvenatives

In Ayurveda many different organ systems will be considered, but for the sake of uniformity I have chosen to focus on the five below to be in keeping with the earlier chapters.

HEART: Saffron, rose, lotus, sandalwood.

SPLEEN: Liquorice, bala.

LUNGS: Elecampane, garlic and fenugreek (taken in milk* with shatavari).

KIDNEYS: Shilajit, brahmi.

LIVER: Aloe gel (with turmeric), barberry (with ghee).

The Kapha Dosha—Dietary recommendations, etc.

The kapha type tends to be slow, tolerant, healthy but with a tendency to excess weight. As water is the predominant element, kapha types may be treated with warming, drying, and reducing therapies (including diuretics, diaphoretics, and emetics). Bitter herbs may be used to reduce sweet cravings. Very few herbs actually increase kapha, so most herbal teas are acceptable, with the avoidance of anything too sweet and mucous forming (e.g., liquorice).

FOODS:

GRAINS: Barley, corn, millet, rye, buckwheat, basmati rice.

BEANS: Mung, red lentils, chickpeas, adzuki. No kidney beans or tofu.

DAIRY: Minimal.

VEG: Onions, cauli, broccoli, radish (mooli), beets, celery, leafy greens.

---

* Personally I would rarely recommend milk as medicine, but in Ayurveda it is considered to be a precious substance. We must also remember that in India the cow is sacred and therefore treated with a great deal more respect than Western cattle. Milk in India is not polluted with hormones and antibiotics and is always taken warm; cold milk is generally not acceptable.

FRUITS: Minimal. Apple, orange peel (as tea or flavouring), pear, cranberry, rosehips (as tea), amla, and schizandra.

SPICES: Black pepper, ginger, bay, coriander, turmeric, fennel, garlic.

MEAT: Minimal. Lamb, chicken, turkey, rabbit.

NUTS: Poppy seeds, sunflower seeds, but NO NUTS.

OILS: Corn, sunflower, but NO NUT OILS.

DRINKS: Tea and other warm drinks before meals, aged wine (in moderation).

Avoid: mucous forming foods, foods that are frozen, processed, sweet, or salty.

DO NOT sleep after eating or eat heavily at night.

The Pitta Dosha—Dietary recommendations, etc.

Because pitta (fire) is naturally hot, the pitta type may be subject to fevers, inflammatory disorders, and a fiery temperament; more cooling, cleansing herbs and foods may be recommended. The pitta diet will be mixed and although primarily cooked will include some raw foods. Hot spices should be avoided, as should the excessive use of oils and stimulants.

MIXED DIET—largely vegetarian

GRAINS: Basmati rice, barley, oats.

PULSES: Avoid beans (except mung and tofu).

DAIRY: Minimal use of dairy (especially cheese).

VEG: Mushrooms, cucumber, squash, asparagus, spinach, potato, carrot, cauli, cabbage, courgette, leafy greens. Avoid tomato and aubergine.

FRUITS: Minimal. Dates, apple, orange, pear, grapes.

MEATS: White meats and white non-oily fish.

SPICES: Coriander, cumin, fennel, turmeric.

DRINKS: Cool drinks (not cold).

OILS: Minimal. Olive, sunflower.

NUTS: None (only seeds such as sunflower).

HERBS: (As teas and decoctions) Alfalfa, burdock, chamomile, chrysanthemum, chicory, coriander, cumin, dandelion, fennel, gotu kola, jasmine, lemon balm, zyziphus, lemon grass, liquorice, marshmallow, sandalwood, skullcap, yellow dock.

Avoid: Foods that are oily, fried, or roasted and salted (e.g., nuts), foods that are sour (e.g., yoghurt), stimulating foods (e.g., coffee, red meat, hot spices, cola).

Pitta types should never eat when irritated, angry, or frustrated.

The Vata Dosha—Dietary recommendations, etc.

Vata (air) is cold, dry, and light; people with this dosha dominating may be fine, brittle, and emotionally sensitive. The major emotion will be fear or anxiety. This type will therefore need warming, nourishing, and "grounding." A building diet of mainly sweet, nourishing foods will usually be recommended.

BUILDING DIET: To nourish blood, skin, hair, and tissues.

GRAIN: Wheat, brown rice, basmati rice.

PULSES: Lentils, kidney beans (fresh), tofu (cooked and well seasoned).

VEGETABLES: All cooked. Onion, garlic, radish, beets, carrots, sweet potatoes, turnip, squash, and asparagus.

FRUITS: Minimal. Dates, cherry, raisins, plums, figs, and lime.

NUTS and SEEDS: Favour almonds, walnuts, and sesame.

SPICES: Ginger, black pepper, anise, coriander, asafoetida.

DRINKS: Warm. Water, teas, diluted fruit juice (lemon, lime, grape).

SILICA RICH FOODS: Alfalfa sprouts, nettle, horsetail.

PUNGENT and SWEET HERBS: As teas or decoctions—not dry powders. Anise, dong quai, cardamom, cinnamon, fo-ti, comfrey, ginger (fresh), gotu kola, rehmania, sarsaparilla, ginseng, and astragalus.

NOURISHING SOUPS: Including lamb, rice, coriander, turmeric, astragalus, ginger, root vegetables, and kelp.

ALMONDS and RICE: Cook blanched almonds and basmati rice together with milk (milk, if tolerated, should be organic; rice milk is a reasonable alternative but not soymilk as it is too cold and stagnating) and jaggery, a very raw and highly nutritious form of sugar. Pound ingredients into a mash when soft—take at least 2 tablespoons, twice daily.

ASTRAGALUS and GINGER: Simmer 20 gm astragalus and 5 gm fresh ginger together in half litre of water for 30 mins, Strain remaining liquid into half pint of milk. Simmer for further 10–15 mins, adding palm sugar or honey to taste (if honey is used, it should be added at end and not cooked).

BREAKFAST: The most important meal for vata types should be warm and cooked, e.g., porridge.

Avoid: Foods that are raw or dry, stimulants (such as coffee, chilli, cola and guarana), eating alone, eating while on the move or watching TV, and fasting.

Key Ayurvedic Formula: *Triphala*

"If you have no mother, but you have Triphala—you'll be okay," is a popular saying in India, where Triphala is considered to be "The mother of all medicines." Triphala does everything that we count on our mother to do; it keeps you clean, it keeps you nourished, and it keeps you regular.

There are, of course, thousands of remedies used by the 5,000-year-old healing tradition of Ayurveda, but the three ingredients of the Triphala formula (harada, amla, bibitaki) will appear in so many of them that to outline the uses and benefits of this simple formula will cover quite a lot of ground.

In the treatment of conditions such as IBS (irritable bowel syndrome), doctor prescribed medicines aim to increase the contraction of gastro-intestinal muscles to aid in creating regular and full bowel movements. Harada (one of the three herbs in Triphala) has been shown to be significantly more effective in achieving this aim than the most commonly prescribed drugs.[18]

Harada (*Haritaki, Terminalia chebula*) is also known as "Buddha's Chosen Herb;" it is sacred amongst Tibetans and shown in the hand of The Medicine Buddha in sacred paintings (*tankas*).

Harada has also been shown to be effective against Helicobacter pylori, the bacteria thought to be responsible for duodenal ulcers[19] and stomach cancer.[20]

Amla (*Indian gooseberry, Emblica officinalis, Phyllanthus Emblica, Amlaki*) is considered to be the richest source of Vitamin C (twenty times that of oranges) making it a valuable source of antioxidants. The high antioxidant tannins in Amla also help to bind the Vitamin C content, making it considerably less viable to loss due to ageing or heating (amla is shown to be heat stable up to 120 degrees centigrade[21]). Amla is also considered to be hepatoprotective.[22]

Behada (*bibitaki, beleric myrobalans, Terminalia belerica*) is both a laxative and astringent, enabling it to clear and tone the bowels; it can therefore be classified as "adaptogenic," as with the other ingredients of Triphala. Behada has antidiabetic, antioxidant, and antimicrobial properties; has potential uses as a remedy for obesity;[23] and has shown to be useful in the treatment of severe conditions such as HIV/AIDS.[24]

Triphala supports the three humours (Tridosha) of Ayurvedic medicine.

Amla, which is cooling, sour, and anti-pyretic, calms the Pitta (fire) humour.

Harada will harmonize the Vata (air) humour, due to its nervine properties.

Behada with its laxative and astringent properties will harmonize the Kapha (earth, water) humour.

Uses: To improve digestion, reduce cholesterol, facilitate circulation, reduce high blood pressure, improve liver function, clear skin and eyes.

Properties: Anti-viral, cardio-protective, anti-oxidant, anti-inflammatory, antidiabetic, anti-microbial, antioxidant.

A problem with many "laxative" medicines (whether pharmaceutical or herbal) is that they can be purging, cooling, and weakening (and in some cases lead to laxative dependency). Whereas Triphala tonifies as it cleanses making it suitable (even for long term use) with most intestinal disorders, including those involving diarrhoea.

CHAPTER TWELVE

East Meets West

AS WITH MY LAST BOOK *100 Herbs of Power* I will devote a small chapter to Middle Eastern Medicine and the work of Avicenna (Abu Ali Ibn Sina 980–1037).

Avicenna was a Persian Scholar and physician who brought together Eastern and Western approaches to healing; he was born in the village of Asfakana, near Bokhara, Greater Persia (now Uzbekistan). Bokhara is on the great Silk Route between Europe and China, a caravan route that has always been a thoroughfare of knowledge, medicines, and merchandise. Bokhara itself was once described as "The Centre of Enlightenment," due to the interchange of cultural and religious ideals.

The Canon of Medicine

Avicenna wrote somewhere in the region of four hundred and fifty treatises on subject matters ranging from astronomy to religion, psychology to physics. The most famous of Avicenna's medical texts is the fourteen-volume classic known as *The Canon of Medicine*, which was completed in the year 1025 A.D.

The Canon discusses a huge amount of medical concepts, including *The Elements, Temperaments and Humours* (all key to "marrying the plants or medicines to the constitution of the patient"). In depth Anatomy, Physiology, and Diagnostic Principles are followed by treatment strategies including liniments, poultices, cupping, bleeding, dietary approaches, and the use of herbs.

Avicenna felt that the body possessed three souls (elsewhere described as "spirits" or "strengths"). The first of these is described as "The Power of Vegetative Actions" or "The Vital Spirit." The Vital Spirit arises within the heart (similar to the concept of "Shen" in Chinese medicine) but is elsewhere described as "breath" (equating it with the Vedic concept of "Prana"). The purpose of The Vital Spirit is to preserve life.

The second of these "Vital Strengths" is described as "The Natural Spirit" or "The Power of Instinct." The Natural Spirit is more animal by nature.* It resides in the Liver and is responsible for growth and reproduction. The third "Vital Strength" is the "Psychic Spirit" or "The Power of Self." The Psychic Spirit resides within the brain and central nervous system; it is rational by nature and responsible for movement and reason.

Avicenna saw disease to be an abnormal state of the body and caused by an imbalance of the humours characterized by blood, phlegm, yellow and black bile. He felt that nature was the great healer and went as far as to say that "many are healed by the actions of nature without the art of medicine," (a concept found also in Ayurvedic medicine and more recently in modern medicine, where a current theory appears to indicate that even tumours may dissipate on their own without medical intervention).

The Materia Medica of Avicenna includes herbs from many cultures such as Agrimony, Chamomile, Elecampane, and Willow Bark from European traditions; Eastern herbs such as Centellia, Asafoetida, and Long Pepper; and of predominantly Middle Eastern plants such as Saffron, Rhubarb Root, and Turmeric. Many mineral and animal medicines were obviously in use also at that time; Avicenna was fond of Pearl Ash, Fullers Earth, beeswax, ambergris, and buttermilk as medicines. Food medicines made a great contribution to Avicenna's healing strat-

---

* In Chinese Medicine The Liver is described as the home of the ethereal soul (Hun) or psychic energy and is often referred to as the tiger or animal spirit.

egies. These included almonds, dates, garlic, and Nigella seeds. Avicenna was the first to distil roses and other plants, and he used these "Attars" or perfume essences, to make up a great deal of his cardiac drugs.

HINDIBA:

> *"Hindiba juice calms the heat of blood and bile and will also benefit the spleen."*
>
> —Isa Efendi

Hindiba was one of Avicenna's tried and tested medicines. It appears to have been derived from Saffron. Cassia fistula was regularly macerated in Hindiba juice as a gargle for tumours and inflammation of the throat.

Ibn al Baitur 1197–1248, the chief herbalist of the King of Egypt, identified Hindiba as having definite anti-cancer properties. Hindiba was patented in 1997 as a cancer drug.

THERIACA:

Avicenna refers a great deal to the compound Theriaca that was originally formulated in first century Greece. Theriaca became popular in both China and India. The legendary history of Theriaca begins with the compound Mithridatium, supposedly formulated by King Mithridates V1 (first century B.C.). King Mithridates was known to be immune to poisons.

Mithridatium contained a high percentage of resins (including frankincense) together with saffron, cinnamon, and around thirty to fifty other herbs. This formula was modified and improved upon by Nero's physician, Andromachus, who brought the number of ingredients up to the alchemical number sixty-four and included viper flesh (pit viper is still used today in Chinese medicine in the treatment of cancer and other "deep-seated" conditions).

The Greek physician Galen devoted an entire book to Theriaca and regularly prescribed it to Marcus Aurelius. The formula took years to gather and prepare, making it extremely expensive. Avicenna considered Theriaca to be a general antidote to snake venom, poisons, and food toxins. This formula was used as a universal panacea until the eighteenth century when it fell out of favour—it would now be considered (at least in Western countries) as not only illegal but also unethical. At least one highly modified Theriaca formula does currently exist in the western world, but it contains very few of the original ingredients.

SAFFRON: (*Zaffran, Kesari,* "bringer of good fortune")

Saffron is used as a powerful medicine by many traditions to treat spiritual, mental, and physical imbalances. It is said to nourish the heart, heighten the spirit, benefit insomnia, aid digestion, act as a sedative, rejuvenative and antidepressant, stimulate menses, and ease labour. Saffron is extremely expensive as it is taken from the tiny stamens of the crocus flower, unfortunately the cheap "saffron" sold in Middle Eastern tourist resorts is usually Safflower, which, although possessing many of saffron's properties, is much milder in action. The best true saffron comes from Kashmir and Iran.

Saffron perfume oil or attar (usually made from blending saffron and sandalwood oils) is delicate, slightly "medicinal" in fragrance, and is considered to be an aphrodisiac.

FRANKINCENSE: (Boswellia Sacra, Boswellia Carteri)

> *"Use frankincense for it invigorates the heart with courage and it is a remedy for forgetfulness."*
> —The Prophet Mohammed

Frankincense was once a key merchandise traded between Rome, Greece, Arabia, China, and India. Pliny recorded that huge amounts was burned by the Emperor Nero at the last rites of his departed wife.

Traditionally frankincense is used to ward off negativity (re exorcism, etc.) and pestilence.

Some of the best frankincense (Hougari) comes from Oman, where it is burned at all festive events. Burned frankincense is a major ingredient in kohl (used as an eye shadow in Eastern countries) and is an ingredient of Theriaca.

The bark of the frankincense tree (in the pine family) can be used, as can the resin. Frankincense oils and attars are also available.

BUKHUR:

A preparation made from agarwood, frankincense, and other woods, roots, barks, and resins, bound in syrup. There are many Bukhur formulae, some dating back 1,000 years.

Origin: Yemen

One of the best Bukhur blends was originally prepared on the highest mountain peak in Yemen and sent throughout Arabia by the Queen of Yemen. Bukhur is used in Islamic holy cities such as Mecca during religious celebrations and is shared with guests as a token of great hospitality. Bukhur is found to aid concentration, improve memory, awaken the mind, enliven the spirit, and repel negative psychic forces.

Although largely used in Islamic ceremonies or by Islamic people, Bukhur is referred to in Christian texts and was used by early Kings of England as an offering (with frankincense and myrrh) at the Feast of Epiphany.

Properties and Uses: Bukhur has been found to be haemostatic, antiseptic, anti-inflammatory, and carminative. Although Bukhur is generally burned on charcoal, it can also be applied to wounds and taken internally (with caution).

Bukhur is found to aid concentration, improve memory, awaken the mind, enliven the spirit, and repel negative forces.

Although normally bought in blocks for burning on charcoal, Bukhur is also available in oil or attar form.

CHAPTER THIRTEEN

The Western Schools

MY FIRST SERIOUS INTEREST IN Herbal Medicine came from the East. As a long-term student of Eastern Philosophy, I found it to be an easy step. I had looked at Western Herbalism and had come to the hasty conclusion that the scars of the Witch Trials still remained, and that the "real meat" of Western Herblore had been long burned out in the fires of The Inquisition. In more recent times I have gained a great respect for many Western herbalists, with whom it has been my privilege to study and work.

As I spend most of my time in the UK, with occasional trips to mainland Europe and the US, I have grown more familiar with the potential of Western botanicals and incorporated hundreds of these into my treatments.

Unfortunately the power of the Church has been replaced by a new religion—Modern Science. And as a result Western Herbal practice is constantly threatened, restricted, and converted to a plant based branch of allopathic medicine, in which herbalists are forced to scientifically verify knowledge, which has already been verified through millennia of traditional use.

So I devote Chapter thirteen (unlucky for some) to many of the great Western Herbalists who have promoted natural medicine, in spite of often-extreme persecution.

In Mediaeval Europe, herbal medicine was only safely practised within the confines of the church, for it was felt that all true healing should come from God or his servants. As a result the monastic tradition produced some great herbalists.

HILDEGARD OF BINGEN: (1098–1179)—"The Sybil of The Rhine"

Hildegard was a Benedictine nun. She was a great visionary, musician, and healer, basing her healing works on the four Humours of Ancient Greek medicine.

Hildegard's two great works on herbal medicine were known as *Physica* and *Causes and Cures* together these texts were called *Liber Subtilatum* (*The Book of Subtleties of the Diverse Nature of Things*).

The sixteenth century was a time of great renaissance in medicine. Throughout Europe Alchemists, Apothecaries, and Herbalists were making their presence felt and, in spite of the inquisition, gaining acceptance and, in some cases, renown.

Dr. John Dee was twice accused of sorcery, and on one occasion charged with plotting to murder Mary Queen of Scots by black magic (via an astrological chart). He was saved from execution due to his friendship with Elizabeth the first and the King of Poland.

Another great physician of that time was the Apothecary and Herbalist of Stratford upon Avon, **Dr. John Hall**, who was the son in law of William Shakespeare and added much to the Herblore in Shakespeare's plays.

The knowledge of Western herbalism, passed down from the time of **Hippocrates** and **Galen**, was later transported to the United States and Canada, where it became influenced by Native American medicine.

European, American, Middle Eastern, Indian, Chinese, and other systems of herbalism continued as separate systems until the twentieth century when the boundaries between them started to dissolve and Western practitioners travelled to China and India to develop their knowledge.

REMBERT DODOENS: (1517–1585)

Dodoens was a Belgian Herbalist and Court Physician of Vienna. He wrote the famous text *Histoire de Plants*. The later *Herbal* or *General History of Plants* by **John Gerard,** included a pirated translation of this text.

NOSTRADAMUS: sixteenth century Apothecary and Seer

Nostradamus is mainly known for his book *The Prophesies*, which first appeared in 1555. He devoted a great deal of his life to occult studies but was also a great herbalist.

After the death of his first wife and their children from the plague, he assisted the great physician **Louis Serre** in treating plague victims. One of the most potent medicines he worked with was made from highly concentrated rose petals.

PARACELSUS: sixteenth century Physician and Alchemist

Although Paracelsus laid the foundations for allopathic and chemical medicine as it is practised today, he as with many "natural physicians" was constantly at loggerheads with exponents of "conventional medicine."

Paracelsus travelled widely throughout Europe and the East, consorting with, and learning from, Romany travellers and Tartar tribesmen. He inspired the development of the highly potentized, alchemically processed, herbal medicines, known as "spagyrics." The preparation of a spagyric essence involves the purifying and recombining of plant components. The aim of the spagyricist is to refine "gold" or "power" from the plant.

NICHOLAS CULPEPPER: seventeenth century Apothecary and Astrologer

Culpepper devoted his life to working with the poor, who could not afford the expensive medicines of the time. He once stated that a major role of the physician was "in the infusion of hope, to induce confidence and peace of mind." He was extremely scathing about the medical profession; he referred to the Royal College of Surgeons as "true vampires." Culpepper was in turn maligned by the College of Physicians for his translation of a Latin Pharmacopoeia into English. His desire to make the knowledge of medicinal plants available to the general public was considered to be some kind of heresy.

Culpepper translated many great texts including those of the second century Greek Physician Galen, emphasizing the importance of the elements of earth, air, fire, and water in maintaining health. Culpepper's own work, in particular his *Complete Herbal* (or *The English Physician*) remains popular today.

SAMUEL THOMPSON: 1769–1843—The Father of American Herbalism.

Samuel Thompson, a former pig farmer, set out to learn natural medicine from studying Native American Herblore. His aim was to replace the medicines used by conventional doctors (the medicines of the day included mercury, arsenic, opium, strychnine, and antimony) with simple herbs including lobelia and cayenne. Thompson was largely responsible for the formation of the "Eclectics" a group, which followed a philosophy of "alignment with nature." Thompson was hounded by the medical profession and taken to court on a trumped up charge of which he was acquitted.

Composition Powder, an aid to both digestion and circulation, was the cornerstone of Thompson's specialized system of herbalism. This combination was not dissimilar in principle to several Ayurvedic formulae (including the digestive formula "Hingashtak" and the Sinus clearing formulae "Trikatu" and "Sitopaladi").

Composition Powder was made famous by another great American Herbalist **Jethro Kloss** (1863–1946), in his best selling book *Back to Eden* and was a favourite formula of **Dr. John Christopher.**

Ingredients of Thompson's Composition Powder:
White Pine (expectorant)
Bayberry (astringent, stimulant)
Cloves (stimulant, anaesthetic, anti-parasitic)
Ginger (stimulates circulation, aids digestion)
Cayenne (pain relieving, diaphoretic)

LYDIA PINKHAM: 1819–1883—"Lily the Pink."

Lydia Pinkham, like Samuel Thompson, was keen to look into the use of natural medicines as alternatives to the both costly

John E. Smith

and toxic medicines prescribed by conventional doctors of her day. She spent many years studying texts such as "John King's American Dispensary" and, like many women of her time, started to brew home remedies. Her remedy for "female complaints" became very popular amongst her friends and eventually led to her son Daniel mass marketing the product in 1876. *Lydia Pinkham's Vegetable Compound* became one of the best-known plant medicines of the nineteenth century. The company continued under the family's control until the 1930s when the FDA (Food and Drug Administration) caused changes in the formula. The compound is now produced by a pharmaceutical company and contains only two of the original ingredients.

A traditional folk song *The Ballad of Lady Pinkham* later became known as an Irish drinking song in which the medicinal compound was described as *"efficacious in every case."* The song was a number one UK hit as *Lily the Pink* (The Scaffold 1968) and a major US hit the year after (The Irish Rovers 1969).

The original formula for Lydia Pinkham's Vegetable Compound contained:
Unicorn Root (known to aid in cases of uterine prolapse)
Life Root (a traditional uterine tonic)
Black Cohosh (traditionally used for menopausal conditions)
Pleurisy Root (an anti-spasmodic herb)
Fenugreek (a known emmenagogue).

BLACK COHOSH—*cimicifuga racemosa*, "black snakeroot."

Actions: Stimulates the uterus (re-delayed menses or labour), promotes cleansing, and helps to antidote poisons.

Uses: Bronchial conditions, high blood pressure, pain, tinnitus, and oestrogen insufficiency.

Cancer Controversies

HARRY HOXSEY:

A herbal cancer medicinal compound was discovered by John Hoxsey in the nineteenth century, while observing the eating habits of a cancer ridden horse whose condition reversed. John Hoxsey's grandson, the naturopath Harry Hoxsey, who later set up cancer clinics throughout the USA, was said to have cured at least twenty five thousand cases of cancer, using the resulting formula.

Professional medical associations and the FDA hounded Harry Hoxsey. He later sued The Journal of the American Medical Association for libel and, although he won the case, the judge only awarded him one dollar in compensation.

The Hoxsey Formula contains:

Red clover blossom, Chaparral herb, Liquorice Root, Buckthorn bark, Burdock root, Stillingia root, Poke root, Barberry root, Oregon grape, Cascara bark, Prickly ash bark, Wild indigo root, and Sea kelp.

RED CLOVER:

Actions: Alterative, diuretic, antibiotic, and anti-inflammatory.

Indications: Cough, skin eruptions, cancer.

Uses: Red clover is blood purifier; it can be used as a paste or salve, for sores that do not heal, or as a gently cleansing tea to clear toxins (including heavy metals). Dissipates tumours (especially in the breasts and ovaries). Benefits the skin and hastens tissue repair. Laboratory tests indicate that red clover has estrogenic and anti-biotic properties.

BURDOCK (*Arctium lappa*)

A majestic plant growing up to six feet high with purple flowering thistle-like burrs.

The root is known in the east as "gobo" and used as a bitter vegetable. Burdock root is often seen in the country markets and specialist stores of Europe. Stir-fried with carrots and other root vegetables, it imparts the bitter flavour so often lacking in western cuisine. In China the seeds are used for treating colds, flu, and throat infections while in the west it is largely the leaf and root that is used externally, as a wash or salve for burns, wounds, and skin irritations. Internally Burdock (often combined with Dandelion) is a good blood cleanser and diuretic, dredging the kidneys, expelling stones, and restraining infection. Burdock is one of the greatest herbs in the treatment of skin conditions.

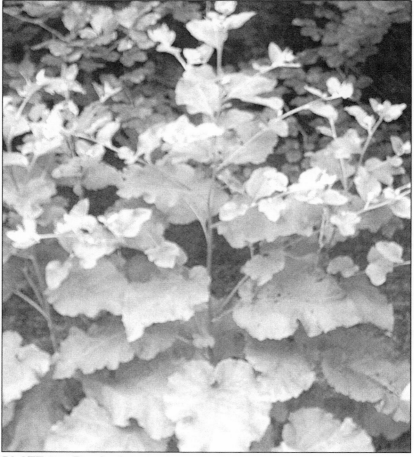

PLATE 6. Burdock.

RENE CAISSE:

The story of Harry Hoxsey is in many ways similar to that of the Canadian nurse Rene Caisse who discovered an herbal formula (which later became known as "Essiac"—"Caisse" spelt backwards), which was used by Ojibwa Indians to treat cancerous disorders.

Rene Caisse did not make a charge for her medicines, and although she was responsible for many cures, she died in relative obscurity after being forced to sell the rights of her formula to the Canadian Health Department for one dollar (the formula was soon "buried").

Caisse Formula (Essiac) contains:
Burdock root, Slippery elm inner bark, Sheep's sorrel, and Indian rhubarb root.

SHEEP'S SORREL (Field Sorrel): (*Rumex acetosella*)

A small edible herb, used in salads and sauces, rich in vitamins and trace elements, particularly silicon. It is necessary for skin, hair, nails, and the nerve-protecting myelin sheath. Sheep's Sorrel is especially relevant as a support herb for the lymphatic system.

Properties: Diuretic, diaphoretic, anti-inflammatory, anti-oxidant.

Uses: Urinary and kidney disorders.

Active ingredients: Phyto-estrogens, glycosides (including quercetin), Vitamins A, B complex, C, D, E, K.

The phyto-estrogens in Sheep's sorrel have a similar oestrogen receptor binding activity, to the isoflavones found in red clover, liquorice, and soya.

History and Folklore: Known as sour grass in Canada where it is used by many indigenous tribes as both food and medicine. Sheep's sorrel was considered the most important herb in *Essiac*, the formula used by Rene Caisse as a cellular regenerative cancer treatment.

Contra-indications: Sheep's Sorrel is very rich in oxalic acid making it unsuitable in high doses for those suffering from kidney stones; oxalic acid is, however, necessary in small amounts for the immune system.

MARIE TREBEN: Austrian Herbalist—1907–1991

As a refugee from Czechoslovakia, Marie Treben contracted Typhoid in a Bavarian Camp. She was introduced to a Swedish Bitters formulation and an ancient document specifying forty-six conditions, which could be treated with the formula. It was thought that Paracelsus produced the original Swedish bitters formula in the sixteenth century.

Marie Treben went on to produce and develop this great formula and applied it with great success to almost every disorder she came across in her work as an herbalist.

Maria Treben was known to have claimed, *"There is a plant for every illness."*

Her first book *Health through God's Pharmacy* sold eight million copies and was translated into twenty-four languages.

The original formula for Swedish bitters contains:

Aloe: Used in cases of stomach ulcers, chronic catarrh, and amenorrhoea.

Myrrh: Stimulant to the mucous tissues, a carminative, exciting the flow of gastric juice.

Saffron: Used for chronic haemorrhage of the uterus in adults.

Senna: Used mainly for severe constipation.

Camphor: Used for colds, chills, and in all inflammatory complaints.

Rhubarb roots: Useful in cases of diarrhoea.

Manna: Thought to be the resin from either a species of Ash (fraxinus orrus) or Tamarisk—Manna is a gentle laxative.

Theriac venezian: (Burnet Saxifrage root) Used for bronchitis, sore throat, indigestion, and catarrh.

Carline thistle roots: Used for bronchitis, headache, inflammation, itchy skin, and kidney stones.

Angelica roots: Used for colds, coughs, pleurisy, wind, colic, and rheumatism.

I have not included many great physicians in my mini biographies, because the list would make a book in itself, as would a list of those practising today. I must, however, acknowledge Christopher Hobbs and Paul Stamets, for their pioneering work with medicinal mushrooms; David Frawley, Vasant Lad, Deepak Chopra, and Sebastian Pole for their clear understanding of Ayurveda; Daniel Reid, Bob Flaws, and Giovanni Maciocia for their presentation of Chinese Herbal strategies; and Michael and Lesley Tierra for bringing much of that knowledge together in Planetary Herbology. And last but not least, for inspiration and courage, Annette Montague Thomas, who, at the time of writing this, is on her eighty-second visit to South Africa, where she is supervising the free herbal care of thousands of HIV/AIDS patients and orphans.[25]

CHAPTER FOURTEEN

Ancient Knowledge and Modern Medicine

THE MAJORITY OF MODERN PHARMACEUTICAL drugs, many of which have been available for no more than a few years, were drawn from plants; seventy-four percent of all drugs contain at least one botanical element.

Whereas pharmaceutical medicine (a relatively new discovery) is generally accepted by the general public, herbal medicine, which has been used been used for thousands of years (and is used, in some form, by eighty percent of The World's population[26]), is still viewed with suspicion by many.

Medicinal plants may (in some cases) contain toxic chemicals, but in most cases other elements in the plant will cushion the effects of these toxins, so that in prescribed doses, even some (not all) quite toxic herbs, will be safe to use. The amount of people harmed from either prescribed or over the counter herb use is rarely worth recording.

When producing a pharmaceutical drug from a plant, the scientist will isolate what is considered to be the "active ingredient" (which in some cases is a toxic alkaloid). This will be analysed in terms of its chemical structure and usually synthesized. In pharmaceutical medicines, the natural plant buffers have been removed, so that all drugs will have at least some side effects. More than two million people suffer damaging side effects each year in the US alone from prescribed medicines and more than

100,000 die from these symptoms.[27] An argument that is often posed is that pharmaceutical medicines go through assiduous trials—this may be true, but it doesn't appear to stop some of the horrendous cases where drugs have to be recalled after a spate of deaths resulting from the use of tested, licensed products.

A scientific theory known as the "uncertainty principle" proposed by the physicist Werner Heisenberg in 1927, states, "the act of observing alters the reality being observed." Although this theory was related to Quantum Physics, I believe that all research will be to some extent, influenced or affected by the researcher—which may mean that we can prove scientifically that science is unscientific (the mind boggles). Claimed research findings may simply measure a prevailing bias among the researchers. How valid is the outcome of herbal research when scientists who are funded by pharmaceutical companies, or the research universities sponsored by them, mainly conduct it?

Herbalists rarely conduct herbal research programs, due to a lack of funding, research facilities, or research skills (or simply a lack of a desire or need to do so). I personally think that scientific tests on herbs are far from conclusive. Herbal medicine is not a science; it is a healing art. Herbs, which have stood the test of time, are traditional remedies not medicinal drugs.

Below is a list of some of the herbs that have been used in the processing of pharmaceutical drugs.

ANDROGRAPHIS Paniculata was used in the production of *Andrographilide* an anti- diarrhoea drug. Both Andrographis and Common Berberis have been used to extract *Berberine*.

CASSIA, a laxative herb, has been used in the drug *Danthron*.

CATARANTHUS (Madagascar Periwinkle) has been used to make two anti-cancer drugs, *Vinblastin* and *Vincristin*.

CHESTNUT (*Aesculus*) has been used in the manufacture of the anti-inflammatory, *Aescin*.

COREOLUS mushroom is used in *PSK* a best selling anti-cancer drug.

CORYDALIS, an herb used in Chinese Medicine to reduce pain, has been used in the analgesic drug *Tetrahydropalmatin*.

DATURA is responsible for the sedative *Scopalamine*.*

EPHEDRA (Mormon Tea)* underlies the antihistamine *Ephedrine*.

GOLDEN SEAL (*Hydrastis*)* is used in the production of *Hydrastine* (an astringent).

KAVA KAVA* (*Piper methysticum*) the Polynesium herb now banned in the EU, has been used to formulate the sedative drug *Kawain*.

LOBELIA INFLATA (Indian Tobacco)* is used in *Lobeline* (a smoking deterrent).

MAYAPPLE (*podophyllum peltatum*) was used in the manufacture of two major cancer drugs, *Etoposide* and *Teniposide*.

MUGWORT, the active constituent of Artemesia annui (sweet wormwood), known as *artemesin,* has been hailed by The World Health Organisation (WHO) as a leading treatment for malaria. *Artemesin* is now used to treat a variety of cancers, including leukaemia, breast, colon, and brain cancer. Mugwort (Artemesia) has been used for thousands of years by Chinese herbalists.

PACIFIC YEW* is used in the manufacture of *Taxol* an anti-tumour drug.

RHODEDENDRON has been used in the tranquilizer *Rhonitoxin*.

SAFFRON. In 1997 an herbal compound for cancer was patented. This formula appeared in Avicenna's "Canon of Medicine" in the tenth century; it was given the name *Hindiba* and appears to be based on the herb saffron.

Another anti-tumour pharmaceutical, *Calchicum*, is also derived from Autumn crocus (saffron).

SARPAGANDHA (*Rauwolfia serpentina*) is used to make the tranquilizer *Rescinnanine* and the circulatory drug *Ajmalicum*.

STEVIA* a natural sweetener was banned in the EU some years ago; it is now used by a pharmaceutical company under the name *Stevioside*.

VALERIAN officinalis has been used in the production of the sedative drug *Valapotriates*.

VINCA MINOR (Lesser Periwinkle) contains an alkaloid known as *vincamine*, which prompts cerebral blood flow, improving the brain's utilization of oxygen and glucose, making this fast growing herb an excellent memory enhancer. *Vinpocetine* is a derivative of *vincamine* and has been used successfully in the treatment of aphasia (loss of the power of speech), mild to moderate dementia apraxia (diminished co-ordination), inner ear problems, and headache. *Vinpocetine* is considered to be a cognitive enhancer, which increases the production of ATP (a cellular energy molecule). *Vinpocetine* is generally regarded as safer than *vincomine* for long term use.

Contra-indications: *Vinpocetine* should not be used if already taking blood thinning medicines such as *warfarin*.

WHITE WILLOW and **MEADOWSWEET** are both rich in salicinic acid, a key ingredient in *Aspirin*. *Salicinic acid* is also used in *Salicin*.

YOHIMBE* an African herb, which has been banned as an over the counter (OTC) product, is used in the aphrodisiac drug *Yohimbine*.

I am definitely not in support of the legalisation of drugs such as cannabis and cocaine, but it would be easy to infer that there is little difference between those pushing drugs on the street and those doing it more openly (except that the latter make a lot more money and are free from prosecution). Take the case of CANNABIS SATIVA (Indian Hemp) as an example. Recently a friendly milkman who was providing cannabis free of charge to arthritic customers was tried in court. The company GW Pharmaceuticals, who produced the Multiple Sclerosis (MS) drug SATIVEX (which is, of course,

---

* The herbs marked with an asterisk are endangered in the wild, restricted, or banned in the EU. It might be interesting to note that the banning of Kava Kava and Stevia, coincided with the development of pharmaceutical products drawn from these plants.

derived from Cannabis Sativa), increased its profits by fifty-one percent.[28]

Regarding COCA, The Bolivian President, Evo Morales, stood up and ate a coca leaf at a recent UN Summit and declared, "This is Coca leaf, it is not cocaine, this is part and parcel of a culture." He told Ministers that the ban on Coca was a "major historical mistake." He added, "It has no harmful impact at all in its natural state. It does not make people run mad, as some would have us believe, and it does not cause addiction." Coca is commonly used in Bolivia and Peru to stave off hunger and altitude sickness, it is also used in cooking. President Morales stated that he was dedicated to tackling the trade in illicit drugs including cocaine.[29]

CHAPTER FIFTEEN

Herbal Alchemy

THERE ARE MEDICINES AND HEALING techniques used by Chinese "energy healers," Tantric Yogis, Tibetan and Mongolian Shaman, and African Sangomas, etc., which defy explanation by either science or "complementary medicine." Alchemy has its links with many of the above traditions, but is also an antecedent of science itself. The alchemist Paracelsus is considered to be "the father of modern medicine," yet he spent much of his life at loggerheads with his own profession, preferring the company of "outsiders" (or what might be referred to today as "practitioners of alternative medicine").

In the modern day alchemical preparations of herbs are produced by advanced practitioners and laboratories throughout the world, using strategies which link Eastern "energetics" with Western science, esoteric and occult principles with those of modern medicine, yet the philosophy of "holism" permeates the entire process.

Alchemical spagyric essences do not take what might be considered to be the active ingredient of an herb and synthesize it (as with modern drug manufacture), but they aim to capture the entire essence of the plant, including its very "soul."

In my own work with herbal medicine, I have recognised that the pharmaceutical approach treats (or suppresses) the symptoms, whereas herbal medicine aims to either prevent the symptom from occurring or treats the underling imbalance, which causes the symptom to be expressed or experienced. However, over the years I have noticed how patients may return after many years of being successfully treated, expressing those same underlying imbalances. It is this that has stimulated my own personal interest in the use of spagyric medicine. Spagyrics set out to not only address the symptoms and underlying imbalances, but also "the cause." The cause may have its origins in childhood, in genetic encoding, or "cellular memories." Some may relate to these causal factors as "past life memories" or simply "inherited traits" or "programmed behavioural tendencies," depending on their ruling philosophy. What really matters in terms of health is that the cause of sickness, whatever it may be, is removed.

Major Figures in the History of Alchemy

HERMES TRISMEGISTUS (Egyptian King 1900 B.C. Contemporary of Moses) Hermes was thought to be the founder of Alchemy. Most of his work was destroyed in the third century A.D. apart from "The Emerald Tablet," which was translated into Arabic by Jabir in the ninth century.

CHANG TAO-LING (The first Taoist Pope. Born 35 A.D.) Received a mystic treatise from Lao Tsu (who had disappeared 500 years previously), which enabled him to manufacture "The Elixir of Life" (or "the nectar of immortality").

JABIR (Arabian Alchemist 721–815 A.D.) Introduced the magic square of the Temple of Light (Ming Tang) brought by Chinese Alchemists via the Silk Route.

AVICENNA (980–1037 A.D.) Author of *The Canon of Medicine* and *The Book of Remedy*. The first person to distil floral essences such as Rose, etc., into the pure, potent perfume/medicines known as **Attars.**

NICHOLAS FLAMEL (fourteenth century) *"Conqueror of the Stone of the Holy Flame"*

"Nicholas" (derived from the Greek meaning
"Conqueror of the Stone")

"Flamel" ("Flam El" = "Holy Flame")

Flamel dreamed of being given a book by an angel. Some time later he stumbled upon a book written by Abraham, which gave details of how the Jews of The Old Testament were saved by turning base metal into gold. It took Flamel many years to decipher the book, and in 1382 he and his wife, Perenelle, succeeded in converting mercury into silver. The following year they were able to convert mercury to gold, and their financial circumstances changed radically, allowing them to donate vast sums to the poor. Nicholas Flamel is thought to have died at the age of 116, after a long period of illness.

PARACELSUS (1493–1540) Rejected accepted medical "knowledge" and preferred to read "nature's books," learning from Romanies and midwives throughout Europe.

Paracelsus was the Founder of "The Doctrine of Signatures," which describes the way nature reveals itself through "signs," e.g., the shape or colour of a plant, etc.

DR. JOHN DEE (1527–1608) Mathematician, Alchemist, Magician, and Court Astrologer. The highly controversial and powerful Dr. John Dee was said to have recorded the "Language of Angels" through Enochian Magic.

During his eventful life he was charged with sorcery on two occasions: once while still at Cambridge for creating a mechanical, flying beetle for a stage play. The second time was in Poland, for claiming to have made a breakthrough in the conversion of lead into gold. Dee was also charged with plotting to murder Mary Queen of Scots, with black magic via an astrological chart. Dee's friendship with Queen Elizabeth the first and the King of Poland, led him to be eventually acquitted of all charges. He died peacefully in Mortlake, the village of his birth, at the age of eighty-one.

COUNT St. GERMAIN (1710–1784) *Sanctus Germanicus,* "Holy Brother." Many rumours exist regarding St. Germain. Some claim him to be "The Wandering Jew" from the time of Christ.

Although Count St. Germain lived during the eighteenth century, he was apparently seen in the late nineteenth century by Annie Besant and again in the twentieth century by H W Leadbeater (both Theosophists). Edgar Cayce ("The Sleeping Prophet") claimed, whilst in a trance, that St. Germain was here "when needed."

It is considered by Theosophists that Count St. Germain has enjoyed many incarnations, including that of Plato, Joseph (husband of Mary), Merlin, Christopher Columbus, and Francis Bacon.

The eighteenth century philosopher Voltaire, referred to Count St. Germain as "A man who never dies, and who knows everything."

St. Germain is best known, in alchemical circles, as the creator of "The Elixir of Life," which was alchemically processed from four substances: Senna, Elderflower, Anise (or possibly Fennel seed), and Manna (Fraxinus ornus—flowering ash).

FULCANELLI (French Alchemist 1920s) Author of *The Mystery of the Cathedrals*—A book in which he suggests that Gothic Cathedrals were alchemical textbooks written in stone, running parallel to the texts relating to The Holy Grail, etc.

Fulcanelli disappeared in the early thirties after performing a transmutation in front of reliable witnesses. He was said to have reappeared several times over the next thirty years looking younger each time. In the 1960s the CIA attempted to track him down, due to his knowledge of nuclear physics. They were unsuccessful.

COUNT CESARE MATTEI (1809–1878) The Creator of "Electro Homeopathy." Mattei was influenced by the works of Paracelsus (Sixteenth century Alchemist) and Hahnemann (the founder of homeopathy). In spite of the ridicule poured upon him by the British medical establishment concerning the claimed success of his cancer cures, Mattei had a huge following in Europe and America, and his work was the subject of more than a hundred publications.

CARL FRIEDRICH ZIMPEL (1800 –1878) A well travelled and learned German Physician and Homeopath. Zimpel was awarded the Prussian gold medal for art and sciences and founded the Zimpel method of Spagyric Essences, now prevalent in Germany, Switzerland, and throughout Europe.

THEODORE KRAUSS (1864–1896) A follower of Count Cesare Mattei. Krauss was largely responsible for the official establishment of spagyric essences in the German Pharmacopeia.

Dr. J GOPALSWAMY NAIDU (born in Mauritius 1958) Dr. Naidu studied chemistry in Russia, gained his Ph.D. in Pharmaceutical Sciences in Switzerland. He continues to produce Spagyric Essences in Switzerland and lectures throughout Europe.

> *"The symptoms of disease are the reason that leads the patient to seek medical help, but his soul and spirit are concealed behind them."*

> *"Illness means a deviation from one's path in life. It is also an opportunity to go back on the right path."*
>
> —Dr. J. G. Naidu

Spagyric Essences

The term "spagyric" comes from two Greek words "spao" (to separate) and "ageiro" (to recombine). The aim of the spagyricist is to unite the principles of body, spirit and soul/sulphur, mercury and salts/alcohol, and essential oils and ash.

There are many stages from harvesting to cohabation (the bringing together of herb elements); they include maceration, filtration, calcination, separation, and purification. In the preparation of a spagyric essence, each stage should take place on the day of the planetary ruler of the herb concerned, e.g., Saturday for herbs governed by Saturn, Sunday for herbs governed by The Sun, etc.

Major Plant Spagyrics Related to Planets

There are many plants related to each planet. I have mentioned just one example per planet in the following list, together with keywords and uses.

SATURN: EQUISETUM (Horsetail)

Keywords: Remineralisation, Lack of affection.

Energetic Level: Stability, to straighten up, gives confidence.

Physical Level: Plant of Kidneys and Bladder (Oedema, Bones, Skin, Osteoporosis). Rich in Silica.

Mental, Emotional: Abnormal fear of injections.

JUPITER: ARNICA

Keywords: To go up, consciousness rising.

Energetic Level: Gives strength to overcome obstacles, gives confidence, hope, new beginnings. Juniper is the plant of becoming.

Physical Level: Remedy for muscles, bruises, sprains, trauma and rheumatic pain.

Mental or emotional: Shock (fast acting remedy with short duration).

MARS: NUX VOMICA

Keywords: Anger, fury, rebelliousness, lack of father's love.

Energetic Level: Stressed, under pressure, allows us to express what's inside, to become positive.

Physical Level: Remedy for the modern man overburdened with responsibility, with unhealthy eating habits. Remedy for excess, hepatic disorders, regulates thyroid.

SUN: EUPHRASIA (eyebright)

Keywords: Awareness, opening, intuition.

Energetic Level: Opens the eyes, to see from the inside, eyes of the soul, third eye, discretion.

Physical Level: Eye problems, hay fever, allergies, hormonal system, and central nervous system.

VENUS: ACHILLEA (Yarrow)

Keywords: Women's liberation, one of the greatest remedies for women.

Energetic Level: Liberation from social customs, e.g., "what will others say." The Shepherd Star announces birth. Brightens chakras. Achillea is a good remedy for beaten women, or men without a female side.

Physical Level: Detoxifying, drains liver/gall, kidneys. Excellent for female hormonal system, for sterility, cysts, fibroids, bruises, bleeding, etc.

MERCURY: MANDRAGORA (Mandrake)

Keywords: Deep sense of life, opening.

Energetic Level: Raped, burned, hanged (even in another life). May relate to a child born with the cord around the neck. Burned taste in mouth, dreams of dragons.

Physical Level: Pain remedy, inflamed large intestine, period pains, painful sex, throat constriction, asthma.

MOON: AGNUS CASTUS

Keywords: Monk's pepper tree

Energetic Level: Psychic castration. For a person who is "mild as a lamb" or unable to say no.

Physical Level: Hormone regulator, "progesterone like." Regulates secretion of mother's milk. Prostate problems—Balances testosterone levels—lack of libido.

John E. Smith

Although in Western Alchemy the plants used in spagyric manufacture are largely Western herbs, the German Pharmacopoeia is gradually expanding as more exotic herbs become included. The Swiss company Phylak, for instance, is producing spagyric essences of Russian Eleutherococcus, Indian Neem, and the African tree Okoubaka.

OKOUBAKA: (*okoubaka aubrevillei*)

Okoubaka is a large tree in the *santalaceae* family. It is mainly found in the West African tropical rain forests. It is used as a "fetish" by African healers to protect against poisonings and ward off evil. The use of Okoubaka is generally restricted to "magicians" and "medicine men."

As a spagyric essence, Okoubaka's keywords include: "The gold of the poor," for detoxification, liberation, and purification. It is considered to be a true remedy for the twenty-first century.

Uses: Okoubaka helps in detoxifying the body from the side effects of pharmaceutical drugs, (including chemotherapy and radio-active iodine), alcohol, coffee, tobacco, and cosmetics. The bark is generally used for treating food poisoning, pesticide poisoning, and other toxic conditions.

Conclusion

IN HERBAL MEDICINE (IN PARTICULAR the Eastern Classical systems), the aim is to make balance. So we tend to treat heat conditions with cooling herbs, which have a calming energy, or cold conditions with more warming, stimulating herbs. There may be some exceptions to this. In China, for instance, it is not uncommon for toxic conditions such as cancer, to be treated successfully with decoctions, including venomous snakes and insects. Homeopathy will also treat "like with like," using untraceable potencies of often poisonous herbs to treat toxic conditions. An underlying rule in natural systems of medicine is that we use nature to treat nature.

Herbal medicines are generally effective, if correctly prescribed, in treating any imbalance, but when that imbalance becomes extremely serious or acute, there may be a place for pharmaceutical medicine or medical procedures.

As mankind moves away from nature and we surround ourselves with man-made causes of disease, the pharmaceutical industries gain greater dominance. But the more we listen to our bodies, eat sensibly, and use natural remedies when appropriate, the healthier we'll remain and the less likely we'll be to take the downward spiral of using unnatural substances to maintain our grip on an unnatural life style.

> *"Pharmaceutical medicine has been used for almost a century to help people to live with their disease, but rarely to cure them."*
> —Professor Hollander, pioneering stem-cell researcher

John E. Smith

*"The Doctor of the future will give no medication,
but will interest his patients in the care of the human
frame, diet and in the cause and prevention of disease."*
                                    —Thomas. A. Edison.

It is my hope that this book will assist my readers in viewing and treating the body as a whole system, rather than as a collection of unrelated parts. And to see our profound, yet delicate, relationship with the world we live in.

Index of Herbs
and Formulae

THERE ARE PROBABLY HUNDREDS OF herbs mentioned in this text, so for this index I have selected only those that have a more detailed profile. I have used the common names of the herbs and formulae, or those more commonly used in the text.

John E. Smith

CHINESE FORMULAE

AYURVEDIC FORMULAE

MIDDLE EASTERN FORMULAE

WESTERN FORMULAE

Bibliography

Appleton, N. *The Curse of Louis Pasteur.*

Avicenna. *The Canon of Medicine.* Adapted by Laleh Bakhtiar, from the translations of Shah/Gruner.

Kazi Publications, Chicago. 1999.

Bensky/Gamble, *Chinese Herbal Medicine 'Materia Medica.'* Eastland Press, Seattle. 1986.

Borhany, Qasi Shaikh Abbas. *Yemen Times,* Issue 863, Volume 13.

Chen, Keji. (Editor), *Imperial Medicaments—Medical Prescriptions Written for Empress Dowager Cixi and Emperor Guangxu with Commentary.* Translated by You Benlin, Foreign Languages Press, Beijing. 1996.

Crow, WB. *The Occult Properties of Herbs.* The Aquarian Press. 1969.

Culpepper, N. *Complete Herbal.* Wordswoth Editions Ltd., 1995.

Davidson, T. *Encyclopedia of Alternative Medicine.*

Fakhirah / Habibullah. *manuscript,* Hiraaz, Yemen.

Fratkin, J. *Chinese Herbal Patent Formulas—A Practical Guide.* Shya Publications, USA. 1986.

Grieve, M. *A Modern Herbal.* Penguin Books. Reprinted 1980.

Gulliver, Peta Jane. *Food Natures Energy Creates You.* Lifeways Publication 1989.

Herbapedia. www.herbnet.com

Hill's Family Herbal. 1812.

John E. Smith

Holmes, Peter. *The Energetics of Western Herbs. Volume 2,* Artemis Press, Colorado. 1989.

Kloss, J. *Back to Eden.* Back to Eden Books, California. 1981 Edition.

Lad/Frawley. *The Yoga of Herbs.*

Maciocia, G. (1989) *The Foundations of Chinese Medicine.* Edinburgh. Churchill Livingstone.

Sams, C. *The Little Food Book.* Alistair Sawday Publishing. 2003.

Smith, J. (Editor) *Planetary Herbals Training Manual*—3rd Edition.

Smith, J. *100 Herbs of Power.* Strategic Book Publishing, New York. 2008.

Stavish, M. *The Path of Alchemy.* Llewellyn Publications, Minnesota. 2006.

Tierra, M. *Guide to Planetary Formulas*—1997.

Tierra, M. *The Wonders of Triphala,* Health Science Institute, May 2002. (From an edited version by John E Smith written for Earthforce UK and The Journal of Complimentary Medicine—with author's consent).

Treben, Maria. *Health through God's Pharmacy.* Ennsthaler, Austria. Second Edition, 1998.

Wikipedia, the free encyclopaedia. www.wikipedia.org/

Glossary of Terms

Adaptogen: A substance, which enables the body to maintain equilibrium

Agni: Hindu god of fire (relates to digestive fire)

AIDS: Acquired Immune Deficiency Disorder

Alchemy: Art of transformation

Ama: Stagnation

Aranyakas: Lit. Forest passages, oral scripture

Arvaryu: Hindu priests responsible for measuring sacrificial ground

Atharva: One of the four main Vedic texts of India

Ayurveda: Indian Science of Life

Brahmanas: Early Vedic texts

Cohabation: The uniting of herb elements

COQ10: An oil soluble, vitamin-like co-enzyme

Dosha: Constitution

EPA: Eicosapentaenoic acid, a nutrient extracted from Omega 3 rich fish oils

GLA: Gamma-linolenic acid, a nutrient extracted from Omega 6 rich seed oils

H5NI: Avian flu virus

HIV: Human Immuno-deficiency Virus

Hotri: Fire priests (Sanskrit)

Hun: Animal or ghost spirits

Itihasas: Myths pertaining to Hindu gods

Jiao: Relates to the three portions of the body, upper, middle, and lower burners

Jing: Essence

Kalonji: Nigella, black seed

Kapha: Earth and water constitution

Kundalini: Serpent power, spinal energy centre

ME: Myalgic Encephalopathy—Chronic Fatigue

Medhya Rasayana: Herbs for the mind

Nasya: Nasal clearing

Pitta: Fire and water constitution

Po: Ministers, Corporeal soul

Qi: Vital Energy

Quercetin: A naturally occurring anti-oxidant, anti-histamine

Rajasic: Stimulating

Ruh: Soul (Arabic)

Samhitas: Lit. collection, referring to Vedic texts

SARS: Severe Acute Respiratory Syndrome

Shen: Spirit (Mandarin)

Soma: Hindu god of the moon, elixir of immortality

Tankas: Sacred pictures (Tibet)

Tridosha: The three constitutions in Ayurveda

Unani Tibb: Lit. Greek Medicine, natural medicine of the Middle East

Upanishads: Vedic Commentaries

Vata: Air and ether constitution

Veda: Wisdom or knowledge, relating to Indian Scripture

Wei Qi: Protective energy

Yang: Outer, expressed energy

Yin: Inner substance

Zhi: Will

Endnotes

1. Marie Nonclerq 1982.
2. See Chapter 9. Rehmania Six formula.
3. The formulae referred to in this paragraph, are manufactured by Planetary Herbals, and are available through major health food stores in the United States.
4. Research study, Kings College, London, 2000.
5. SHEN or Spirit, which refers to an immortal energy (sometimes referred to as "The Messengers of Heaven"). Shen is said to remain eternally after the death of the body.
6. THE 7 PO or Ministers, return to the earth as metal at the body's demise.
7. THE 3 HUN, Animal or Ghost spirits: these are said to continue for three generations after the death of the body.
8. Ghirlanda G, Oradei A, Manto A, Lippa S, Uccioli L, Caputo S, Greco A, Littarru G (1993). "Evidence of plasma CoQ10-lowering effect by HMG-CoA reductase inhibitors: a double-blind, placebo-controlled study." *J Clin Pharmacol* 33 (3): 226–9.
9. M. Berdoy, J. P. Webster and D. W. Macdonald. "Fatal attraction in rats infected with Toxoplasma gondi." Proc Biol Sci 2000.
10. M. Manal 1930.
11. Dr. J. Naidu. Phylak Spagyricist.
12. Adaptogenic: enables the body to withstand stress, and regain, or maintain, a state of balance.
13. Rode, Dorena "Summary of In Vivo Comfrey Studies" Retrieved Feb. 2008.
14. Moerman 1998, Reina-Guerren 1993, Yetman & Fulger 2002.

15. Bensky and Gamble 1993.
16. *Herbalpedia.* www.herbnet.com and *Wikipedia.*
17. The moon is thought to represent Soma or ambrosia. Ambrosia, Ambrotus, and Amrita (non-dead, water of life) are at the root of the word "immortality." In Vedic myth "ambrosia" is described as "Soma." Some say that Soma referred to the juice of a climbing plant (now presumably extinct), which endowed immortality and poetic inspiration. Others connect it to various plants from fly agaric to cannabis sativa, from ginkgo biloba to ephedra.

    Soma is also known as Chandra and identified in Hinduism as the Moon. The god Chandra (Soma) was produced from the churning of the milk ocean. He was considered to be the brother of the goddess Lakshmi (also born from the milk ocean). Soma fathered Gautama through Tara (the wife of Brihaspati) and was banished to the outer realms by Brahma.
18. Tamhane M D, Thorat S P. Rege N N, Dahanukar S A, Effect of oral administration of Terminalia chebula on gastric emptying: an experimental study. J.Postgrad Med 1997 Jan–Mar; 43(1) : 12-3.
19. Malekzadeh F, Ensanifar H, Shahamat M, Levin M, Colwell R R. Antibacterial activity of black Myrobalans (Terminalia chebula Retz) against Helicobacter pylori. Int J Antimicrob Agents 2001 July; 18(1): 85-8.
20. K. Tokura and S. Kagawa, "Anticancer agents containing chebulanin from Terminalia chebula," Jpn. Kokai Tokkyo Koho JP 07,138,165, Sept. 24th, 1995.
21. A study on degradation kinetics of ascorbic acid in amla (Phyllanthus Emblica L.) during cooking. Int J Food Sci Nutri. 2004 Aug; 55(5): 415-22.
22. R. Gulati, S. Agarwal and S.S. Agarwal, "Hepatoprotective studies on Phyllanthus Emblica and Quercetin." Indian J. Exp. Biol. 33(4), 261-268, 1995.
23. M. Hashimoto and Y. Nakajima, "Antiobesity agents, alpha-amalase inhibitors, lipase inhibitors, foods and beverages

containing plant extracts" Jpn, Kokai Tokkyo Koho JP 09, 227, 398, 2/9/97.

24. T. Hozumi, H. Oyama et al., "Crude drugs for treating AIDS" Jpn. Kokai Tokkyo Koho JP 09 87, 185, 1997.
25. For information on Annette's work contact The Global Natural Healthcare Trust—www.gnhct.org.
26. World Health Organisation.
27. Journal of the American Medical Association, Volume 279 No. 15, April 15th 1998.
28. The Independent. Thursday 12th March 2009.
29. The Independent. Thursday 12th March 2009.

Lightning Source UK Ltd.
Milton Keynes UK
23 March 2010
151801UK00001B/17/P